Radiography and
Radiology for Dental Nurses

Dedication
To Catriona, Stuart, Felicity and Claudia

Commissioning Editor: Michael Parkinson
Project Development Manager: Clive Hewat
Project Manager: David Fleming
Designer: Erik Bigland

Radiography and Radiology for Dental Nurses

WRITTEN AND ILLUSTRATED BY

Eric Whaites

MSc BDS(Hons) FDSRCS(Edin) FDSRCS(Eng) FRCR DDRRCR

Senior Lecturer and Honorary Consultant in Dental Radiology and Head of the Department of Dental Radiology, Guy's, King's and St Thomas' Dental Institute, King's College London, London, UK

FOREWORD BY

Diana Wincott MBE

Head of the Guy's, King's and St Thomas' Dental Nurse Education and Training Centre

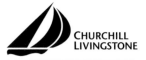

CHURCHILL
LIVINGSTONE

EDINBURGH LONDON NEW YORK OXFORD PHILADELPHIA ST LOUIS SYDNEY TORONTO 2005

ELSEVIER | CHURCHILL LIVINGSTONE
An imprint of Elsevier Limited

First published 2005

ISBN 0-443-10213 9

British Library Cataloguing in Publication Data
A catalogue record for this book is available from the British Library

Library of Congress Cataloging in Publication Data
A catalog record for this book is available from the Library of Congress

Notice
Medical knowledge is constantly changing. Standard safety precautions must be followed, but as new research and clinical experience broaden our knowledge, changes in treatment and drug therapy may become necessary or appropriate. Readers are advised to check the most current product information provided by the manufacturer of each drug to be administered to verify the recommended dose, the method and duration of administration, and contraindications. It is the responsibility of the practitioner, relying on experience and knowledge of the patient, to determine dosages and the best treatment for each individual patient. Neither the Publisher nor the author assumes any liability for any injury and/or damage to persons or property arising from this publication.

The Publisher

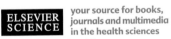
your source for books, journals and multimedia in the health sciences

www.elsevierhealth.com

The publisher's policy is to use **paper manufactured from sustainable forests**

Printed in China

Contents

Foreword

I am delighted to have been asked to write the Foreword and lend my support to a textbook which has been specifically edited for Dental Nurses. The timely publication of Eric Whaites' book, which is based on his well established 'Essentials of Dental Radiography and Radiology', will go a long way to support learners and provide, for the first time, a significant reference text suitable for all Professions Complimentary to Dentistry.

A national certificate allowing qualified Dental Nurses to take dental radiographs in the UK has been in demand, by dentists and dental nurses alike, for a number of years now. Such a certificate has now been developed by the National Examining Board for Dental Nurses in partnership with the British Society of Dental and Maxillofacial Radiology, the College of Radiographers and the British Dental Association. I believe this book which offers a clear, easy to follow, comprehensive account of all aspects of dental radiography that are relevant to dental nurses will become an important resource to students and trainers alike and expect it to be become essential reading for those undertaking this new Certificate in Dental Radiography.

Diana Wincott MBE
Head of the Guy's, King's and St Thomas' Dental Nurse Education & Training Centre

Preface

The aim of my original 'Essentials of Dental Radiography and Radiology' was to provide a basic and practical account of what I considered to be the essential subject matter of both dental radiography and radiology for undergraduate and postgraduate dental students, as well as for students of the Professions Complimentary to Dentistry (PCDs). The main target audience has undoubtedly been undergraduate dental students. Whilst many PCDs, including dental nurses, have utilised this book over the years, it is apparent that the section on radiological interpretation was largely irrelevant to them.

It seemed prudent therefore to produce a condensed version of the dental student book intended specifically for dental nurses. Judicious editing has hopefully ensured that the resultant package is comprehensive and concentrates on relevant topics. I have not attempted to re-write the text.

Some radiological interpretation remains, particularly of the teeth and their supporting structures and I have included an atlas style chapter showing examples of some of the more important abnormal conditions that dental nurses may observe in the clinical setting.

This version remains first and foremost a teaching manual, rather than a comprehensive reference book. I hope the content remains sufficiently detailed and broad to satisfy the requirements of most post-qualification certificate examinations for dental nurses.

I have endeavoured to make a positive contribution to the challenging task facing dental nurses as they embark on broadening their careers to include dental radiography.

EJW
2004

Acknowledgements

The impetus for this shortened version of my dental student 'Essentials' book, aimed specifically at dental nurses, came from four people from the National Examining Board for Dental Nurses (NEBDN) namely David Craig, Jennifer Lavery, Janet Goodwin and James Mehta. I am extremely grateful for their enthusiasim for this venture, to support the training of dental nurses in dental radiography.

However, this edition for dental nurses has only been possible because of the enormous amount of help and encouragement that I received from my family, friends and colleagues that allowed me to produce the third edition of 'Essentials' for dental students, upon which this book is based. I would therefore, once again, like to thank the members of staff in my Department, both past and present, particularly Mrs Jackie Brown, Mr Nicholas Drage, Mr Brian O'Riordan, Professor David Smith, Mrs Nadine White, Ms Jocelyn Sewell, Ms Sharon Duncan and Miss Allisson Summerfield for their collective help and encouragement. As I have said before, I am indeed fortunate to work with, and have worked with, such an able and supportive team.

My thanks to the following for their help and advice with specific chapters: Dr Neil Lewis (Chapter 6), Mr Peter Hirschmann, Mr Tony Hudson, Mr Ian Napier and the NRPB for allowing me to reproduce parts of the 2001 Guidance Notes (Chapter 6), Mr Guy Palmer and Dr Carole Boyle (Chapter 7), Professor Fraser Macdonald (Chapter 12), Mr Sohaib Safiullah (Chapter 20), Professor Richard Palmer (Chapter 21). My thanks also to the many colleagues and students who have provided comments and feedback over the years that I hope have led to improvements.

Special thanks to Mr Ted Dawson, Mr Andrew Dyer and Mrs Emma Wing of the GKT Department of Photography, Printing and Design who spent so many hours producing the clinical photographs and radiographic illustrations which are so crucial to a book that relies heavily on visual images. My thanks also to Miss Julie Cooper for willingly sitting as the photographic model.

My thanks also to Mr Clive Hewat and the staff of Elsevier for their help and advice in the production process.

It is easy to forget the help provided with the initial 'Essentials' manuscript several years ago, but without the help of Professor Rod Cawson this book would never have been produced in the first place. My thanks once again to him and to my various colleagues who have helped me over the years.

Introduction

1 The radiographic image

Introduction

The use of X-rays is an integral part of clinical dentistry, with some form of radiographic examination necessary on the majority of patients. As a result, radiographs are often referred to as the clinician's *main diagnostic aid*.

The range of knowledge of dental radiography and radiology thus required can be divided conveniently into four main sections:

- *Basic physics and equipment* — the production of X-rays, their properties and interactions which result in the formation of the radiographic image
- *Radiation protection* — the protection of patients and dental staff from the harmful effects of X-rays
- *Radiography* — the techniques involved in producing the various radiographic images
- *Radiology* — the interpretation of these radiographic images.

Understanding the radiographic image is central to the entire subject. This chapter provides an introduction to the nature of this image and to some of the factors that affect its quality and perception.

Nature of the radiographic image

The image is produced by X-rays passing through an object and interacting with the photographic emulsion on a film. This interaction results in blackening of the film. The extent to which the emulsion is blackened depends on the number of X-rays reaching the film, which in turn depends on the density of the object.

The final image can be described as a two-dimensional picture made up of a variety of black, white and grey superimposed shadows and is thus sometimes referred to as a *shadowgraph* (see Fig. 1.1).

Understanding the nature of the shadowgraph and interpreting the information contained within it requires a knowledge of:

- The radiographic shadows
- The three-dimensional anatomical tissues
- The limitations imposed by a two-dimensional picture and superimposition.

The radiographic shadows

The amount the X-ray beam is stopped (attenuated) by an object determines the *radiodensity* of the shadows:

- The white or *radiopaque* shadows on a film represent the various dense structures within the object which have totally stopped the X-ray beam.
- The black or *radiolucent* shadows represent areas where the X-ray beam has passed through the object and has not been stopped at all.
- The grey shadows represent areas where the X-ray beam has been stopped to a varying degree.

The final *shadow density* of any object is thus affected by:

- The specific type of material of which the object is made
- The thickness or density of the material
- The shape of the object
- The intensity of the X-ray beam used

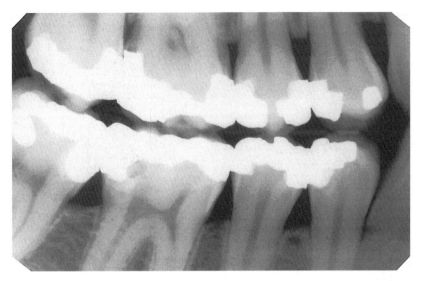

Fig. 1.1 A typical dental radiograph. The image shows the various black, grey and white radiographic shadows.

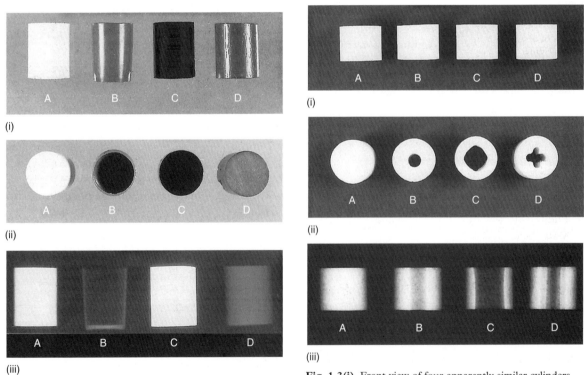

Fig. 1.2(i) Front view and **(ii)** plan view of various cylinders of similar shape but made of different materials: **A** plaster of Paris, **B** hollow plastic, **C** metal, **D** wood. **(iii)** Radiographs of the cylinders show how objects of the same shape, but of different materials, produce different radiographic images.

Fig. 1.3(i) Front view of four apparently similar cylinders made from plaster of Paris. **(ii)** Plan view shows the cylinders have varying internal designs and thicknesses. **(iii)** Radiographs of the apparently similar cylinders show how objects of similar shape and material, but of different densities, produce different radiographic images.

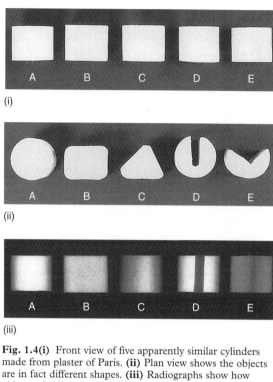

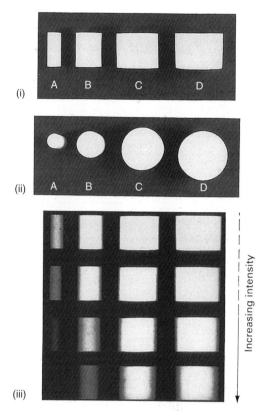

Fig. 1.4(i) Front view of five apparently similar cylinders made from plaster of Paris. **(ii)** Plan view shows the objects are in fact different shapes. **(iii)** Radiographs show how objects of different shape, but made of the same material, produce different radiographic images.

Fig. 1.5(i) Front view and **(ii)** plan view of four cylinders made from plaster of Paris but of different diameters. **(iii)** Four radiographs using different intensity X-ray beams show how increasing the intensity of the X-ray beam causes greater penetration of the object with less attenuation, hence the less radiopaque (white) shadows of the object that are produced, particularly of the smallest cylinder.

- The position of the object in relation to the X-ray beam and film
- The sensitivity of the film.

The effect of different materials, different thicknesses/densities, different shapes and different X-ray beam intensities on the radiographic image shadows are shown in Figures 1.2–1.5.

The three-dimensional anatomical tissues

The shape, density and thickness of the patient's tissues, principally the hard tissues, must also affect the radiographic image. Therefore, when viewing two-dimensional radiographic images, the three-dimensional anatomy responsible for the image must be considered (see Fig. 1.6). A sound anatomical knowledge is obviously a prerequisite for radiological interpretation (see Ch. 18).

The limitations imposed by a two-dimensional image and superimposition

The main limitations of viewing the two-dimensional image of a three-dimensional object are:

- Appreciating the overall shape of the object
- Superimposition and assessing the location and shape of structures *within* an object.

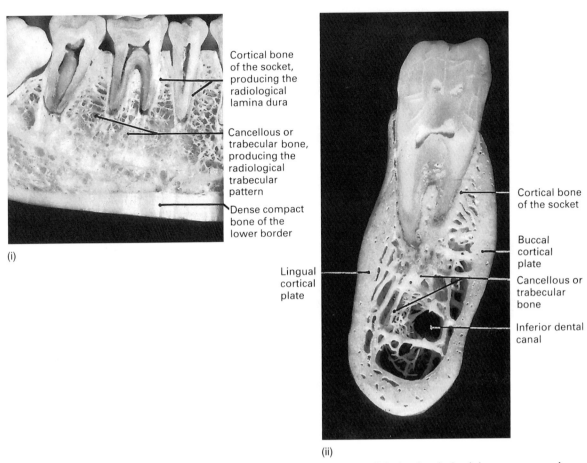

Cortical bone
of the socket,
producing the
radiological
lamina dura

Cancellous or
trabecular bone,
producing the
radiological
trabecular
pattern

Dense compact
bone of the
lower border

(i)

Cortical bone
of the socket

Buccal
cortical
plate

Cancellous or
trabecular
bone

Inferior dental
canal

Lingual
cortical
plate

(ii)

Fig. 1.6A **(i)** Sagittal and **(ii)** coronal sections through the body of a dried mandible showing the hard tissue anatomy and internal bone pattern.

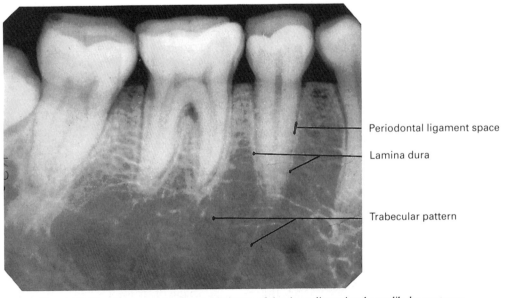

Periodontal ligament space

Lamina dura

Trabecular pattern

Fig. 1.6B Two-dimensional radiographic image of the three-dimensional mandibular anatomy.

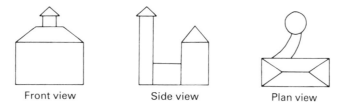

Front view   Side view   Plan view

Fig. 1.7 Diagram illustrating three views of a house. The side view shows that there is a corridor at the back of the house leading to a tall tower. The plan view provides the additional pieces of information that the roof of the tall tower is round and that the corridor is curved.

Appreciating the overall shape

To visualize all aspects of any three-dimensional object, it must be viewed from several different positions. This can be illustrated by considering an object such as a *house*, and the minimum information required if an architect is to draw all aspects of the three-dimensional building in two dimensions (see Fig. 1.7). Unfortunately, it is only too easy for the observer to forget that teeth and patients are three-dimensional. To expect one radiograph to provide *all* the required information about the shape of a tooth or patient is like asking

the architect to describe the whole house from the front view alone.

Superimposition and assessing the location and shape of structures within an object

The shadows cast by different parts of an object (or patient) are superimposed upon one another on the final radiograph. The image therefore provides limited or even misleading information as to where a particular internal structure lies, or to its shape, as shown in Figure 1.8.

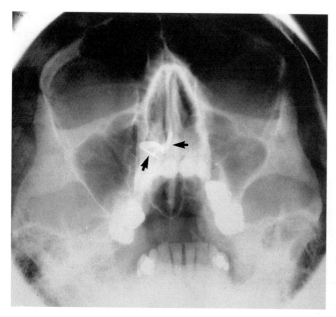

Fig. 1.8 Radiograph of the head from the front (an *occipitomental* view) taken with the head tipped back, as described later in Chapter 12. This positioning lowers the dense bones of the base of the skull and raises the facial bones so avoiding superimposition of one on the other. A radiopaque (white) object (arrowed) can be seen apparently in the base of the right nasal cavity.

In addition, a dense radiopaque shadow on one side of the head may overlie an area of radiolucency on the other, so obscuring it from view, or a radiolucent shadow may make a superimposed radiopaque shadow appear less opaque. One clinical solution to these problems is to take two views, at right angles to one another (see Figs 1.9 and 1.10). Unfortunately, even two views may still not be able to provide all the desired information for a diagnosis to be made (see Fig. 1.11).

These limitations of the conventional radiographic image have very important clinical implications and may be the underlying reason for a *negative radiographic report*. The fact that a particular feature or condition is not visible on one radiograph does not mean that the feature or condition does not exist, merely that it cannot be seen. Many of the recently developed alternative and specialized imaging modalities such as CT and MRI have been designed to try to overcome these limitations.

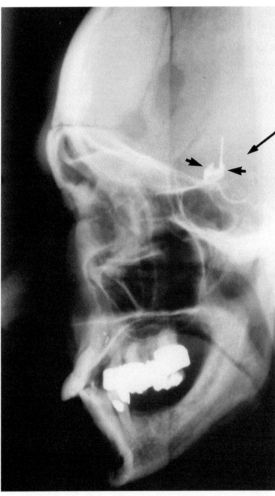

Fig. 1.9 Radiograph of the head from the side (a *true lateral skull view*) of the same patient shown in Figure 1.8. The radiopaque (white) object (arrowed) now appears intracranially just above the skull base. It is in fact a metallic aneurysm clip positioned on an artery in the Circle of Willis at the base of the brain. The dotted line indicates the direction of the X-ray beam required to produce the radiograph in Figure 1.8, illustrating how an intracranial metallic clip can appear to be in the nose.

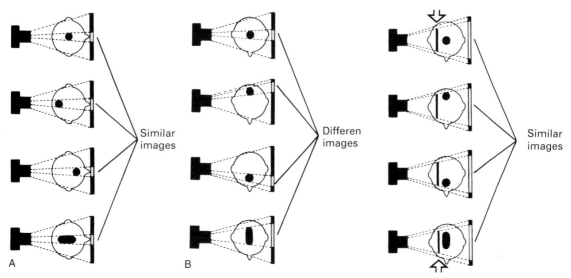

Fig. 1.10 Diagrams illustrating the limitations of a two-dimensional image: **A** Postero-anterior views of a head containing a mass in a different position or of a different shape. In all the examples, the mass will appear as a similar sized opaque image on the radiograph, providing no differentiating information on its position or shape. **B** The lateral or side view provides a possible solution to the problems illustrated in **A**; the masses now produce different images.

Fig. 1.11 Diagrams illustrating the problems of superimposition. Lateral views of the same masses shown in Figure 1.10 but with an additional radiodense object superimposed. This produces a similar image in each case with no evidence of the mass. The information obtained previously is now obscured and the usefulness of using two views at right angles is negated.

Quality of the radiographic image

Overall image quality and the amount of detail shown on a radiograph depend on several factors, including:

- Contrast — the visual difference between the various black, white and grey shadows
- Image geometry — the relative positions of the film, object and X-ray tubehead
- Characteristics of the X-ray beam
- Image sharpness and resolution.

These factors are in turn dependent on several variables, relating to the density of the object, the image receptor and the X-ray equipment. They are discussed in greater detail in Chapter 15. However, to introduce how the geometrical accuracy and detail of the final image can be influenced, two of the main factors are considered below.

Positioning of the film, object and X-ray beam

The position of the X-ray beam, object and film needs to satisfy certain basic geometrical requirements. These include:

- The object and the film should be in contact or as close together as possible
- The object and the film should be parallel to one another
- The X-ray tubehead should be positioned so that the beam meets both the object and the film at right angles.

These ideal requirements are shown diagrammatically in Figure 1.12. The effects on the final image of varying the position of the object, film or X-ray beam are shown in Figure 1.13.

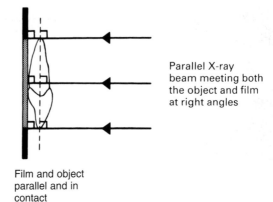

Parallel X-ray beam meeting both the object and film at right angles

Film and object parallel and in contact

Fig. 1.12 Diagram illustrating the ideal geometrical relationship between the film, object and X-ray beam.

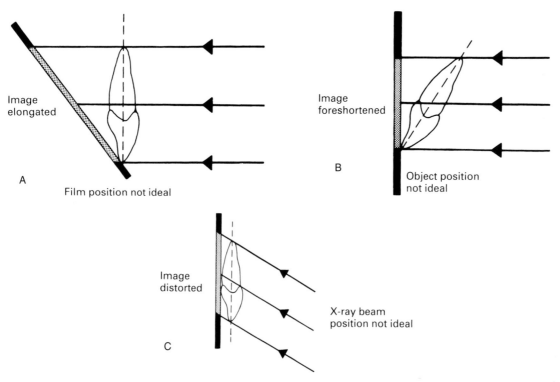

Image elongated

A

Film position not ideal

Image foreshortened

B

Object position not ideal

Image distorted

X-ray beam position not ideal

C

Fig. 1.13 Diagrams showing the effect on the final image of varying the position of **A** the film, **B** the object and **C** the X-ray beam.

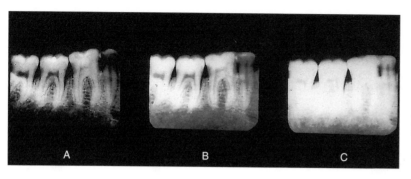

Fig. 1.14 Radiographs of the same area showing variation in contrast — the visual difference in the black, white and grey shadows due to the penetration of the X-ray beam. **A** Increased exposure (overpenetration). **B** Normal exposure. **C** Reduced exposure (underpenetration).

X-ray beam characteristics

The ideal X-ray beam used for imaging should be:

- Sufficiently penetrating, to pass through the patient and react with the film emulsion and produce good *contrast* between the different shadows (Fig. 1.14)
- Parallel, i.e. non-diverging, to prevent magnification of the image
- Produced from a point source, to reduce blurring of the edges of the image, a phenomenon known as the *penumbra* effect.

These ideal characteristics are discussed further in Chapter 5.

Perception of the radiographic image

The verb *to perceive* means *to apprehend with the mind using one or more of the senses*. Perception is the *act* or *faculty of perceiving*. In radiology, we use our sense of sight to perceive the radiographic image, but, unfortunately, we cannot rely completely on what we see. The apparently simple black, white and grey shadowgraph is a form of optical *illusion* (from the Latin *illudere*, meaning *to mock*). The radiographic image can thus mock our senses in a number of ways. The main problems can be caused by the effects of:

- Partial images
- Contrast
- Context.

Effect of partial images

As mentioned already, the radiographic image only provides the clinician with a partial image with limited information in the form of different density shadows. To complete the picture, the clinician fills in the gaps, but we do not all necessarily do this in the same way and may arrive at different conclusions. Three non-clinical examples are shown in Figure 1.15. Clinically, our differing perceptions may lead to different diagnoses.

Effect of contrast

The apparent density of a particular radiographic shadow can be affected considerably by the density of the surrounding shadows. In other words, the contrast between adjacent structures can alter the perceived density of one or both of them (see Fig. 1.16). This is of particular importance in dentistry, where metallic restorations produce densely white radiopaque shadows that can affect the apparent density of the adjacent tooth tissue. This is discussed again in Chapter 18 in relation to caries diagnosis.

Effect of context

The environment or context in which we see an image can affect how we interpret that image. A non-clinical example is shown in Figure 1.17. In dentistry, the environment that can affect our perception of radiographs is that created by the patient's description of the complaint. We can imagine that we see certain radiographic changes, because the patient has conditioned our perceptual apparatus.

These various perceptual problems are included simply as a warning that radiographic interpretation is not as straightforward as it may at first appear.

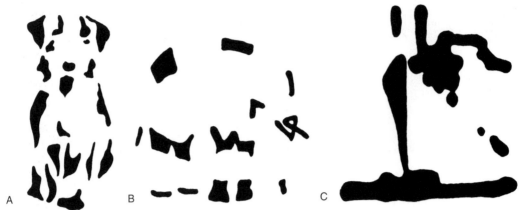

A   B   C

Fig. 1.15 The problem of partial images requiring the observer to fill in the missing gaps. Look at the three non-clinical pictures and what do you perceive? The objects shown are **A** a dog, **B** an elephant and **C** a steam ship. We all *see* the same partial images, but we don't necessarily *perceive* the same objects. Most people perceive the dog, some perceive the elephant while only a few perceive the ship and take some convincing that it is there. Interestingly, once observers have perceived the correct objects, it is impossible to look at the pictures again in the future without perceiving them correctly. (Figures from: Coren S, Porac C, Ward LM 1979 Sensation and perception. Harcourt Brace and Company, reproduced by permission of the publisher.)

Fig. 1.16 The effect of contrast. The four small inner squares are in reality all the same grey colour, but they appear to be different because of the effect of contrast. When the surrounding square is black, the observer perceives the inner square to be very pale, while when the surrounding square is light grey, the observer perceives the inner square to be dark. (Figure from: Cornsweet TN 1970 Visual perception. Harcourt Brace and Company, reproduced by permission of the publisher.)

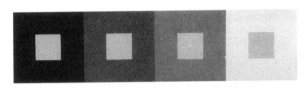

Fig. 1.17 The effect of context. If asked to read the two lines shown here most, if not all, observers would read the letters A,B,C,D,E,F and then the numbers 10,11,12,13,14. Closer examination shows the letter B and the number 13 to be identical. They are perceived as B and 13 because of the context (surrounding letters or numbers) in which they are seen. (Figure from: Coren S, Porac C, Ward LM 1979 Sensation and perception. Harcourt Brace and Company, reproduced by permission of the publisher.)

Common types of dental radiographs

The various radiographic images of the teeth, jaws and skull are divided into two main groups:

- *Intraoral* — the film is placed *inside* the patient's mouth, including:
  - Periapical radiographs (Ch. 8)
  - Bitewing radiographs (Ch. 9)
  - Occlusal radiographs (Ch. 10)
- *Extraoral* — the film is placed *outside* the patient's mouth, including:
  - Oblique lateral radiographs (Ch. 11)
  - Lateral skull radiographs (Ch 12)
  - Dental panoramic tomographs (Ch. 13).

These various radiographic techniques are described later, in the chapters indicated. The approach and format adopted throughout these radiography chapters are intended to be straightforward, practical and clinically relevant and are based upon the essential knowledge required. This includes:

- WHY each particular projection is taken — i.e. the main clinical indications
- HOW the projections are taken — i.e. the relative positions of the patient, film and X-ray tubehead
- WHAT the resultant radiographs should look like and which anatomical features they show.

Radiation physics and equipment

Part
2

2 The production, properties and interactions of X-rays

Introduction

X-rays and their ability to penetrate human tissues were discovered by Roentgen in 1895. He called them X-rays because their nature was then unknown. They are in fact a form of high-energy electromagnetic radiation and are part of the electromagnetic spectrum, which also includes low-energy radiowaves, television and visible light (see Table 2.1).

X-rays are described as consisting of *wave packets* of energy. Each packet is called *a photon* and is equivalent to one *quantum* of energy. The X-ray *beam*, as used in diagnostic radiology, is made up of millions of individual photons.

To understand the production and interactions of X-rays a basic knowledge of atomic physics is essential. The next section aims to provide a simple summary of this required background information.

Atomic structure

Atoms are the basic building blocks of matter. They consist of minute particles — the so-called fundamental or elementary particles — held together by electric and nuclear forces. They consist of a central dense *nucleus* made up of nuclear particles — *protons* and *neutrons* — surrounded by *electrons* in specific orbits or shells (see Fig. 2.1).

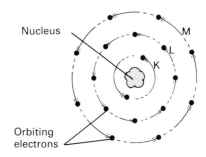

Fig. 2.1 Diagrammatic representation of atomic structure showing the central nucleus and orbiting electrons.

Table 2.1 The electromagnetic spectrum ranging from the low energy (long wavelength) radio waves to the high energy (short wavelength) X- and gamma-rays

Radiation	Wavelength	Photon energy
Radio, television and radar waves	3×10^4 m to 100 µm	4.1×10^{-11} eV to 1.2×10^{-2} eV
Infra-red	100 µm to 700 nm	1.2×10^{-2} eV to 1.8 eV
Visible light	700 nm to 400 nm	1.8 eV to 3.1 eV
Ultra-violet	400 nm to 10 nm	3.1 eV to 124 eV
X- and gamma-rays	10 nm to 0.01 pm	124 eV to 124 MeV

Useful definitions

- *Atomic number* (Z) — The number of protons in the nucleus of an atom
- *Neutron number* (N) — The number of neutrons in the nucleus of an atom
- *Atomic mass number* (A) — Sum of the number of protons and number of neutrons in an atom (A = Z + N)
- *Isotopes* — Atoms with the same atomic number (Z) but with different atomic mass numbers (A) and hence different numbers of neutrons (N)
- *Radioisotopes* — Isotopes with unstable nuclei which undergo radioactive disintegration.

Main features of the atomic particles

Nuclear particles (nucleons)

Protons

- Mass = 1.66×10^{-27} kg
- Charge = positive: 1.6×10^{-19} coulombs.

Neutrons

- Mass = 1.70×10^{-27} kg
- Charge = nil
- Neutrons act as *binding agents* within the nucleus and hold it together by counteracting the repulsive forces between the protons.

Electrons

- Mass = 1/1840 of the mass of a proton
- Charge = negative: -1.6×10^{-19} coulombs
- Electrons move in predetermined circular or elliptical shells or orbits around the nucleus
- The shells represent different *energy levels* and are labelled K,L,M,N,O outwards from the nucleus
- The shells can contain up to a maximum number of electrons per shell:
    - K ... 2
    - L ... 8
    - M ... 18
    - N ... 32
    - O ... 50
- Electrons can move from shell to shell but cannot exist between shells — an area known as the *forbidden zone*
- To remove an electron from the atom, additional energy is required to overcome the *binding energy* of attraction which keeps the electrons in their shells.

Summary of important points on atomic structure

- In the neutral atom, the number of orbiting electrons is equal to the number of protons in the nucleus. Since the number of electrons determines the chemical behaviour of an atom, the *atomic number* (Z) also determines this chemical behaviour. Each *element* has different chemical properties and thus each *element* has a different *atomic number*. These form the basis of the *periodic table*.
- Atoms in the ground state are electrically neutral because the number of positive charges (protons) is balanced by the number of negative charges (electrons).
- If an electron is removed, the atom is no longer neutral, but becomes positively charged and is referred to as a *positive ion*. The process of removing an electron from an atom is called *ionization*.
- If an electron is displaced from an inner shell to an outer shell (i.e. to a higher energy level), the atom remains neutral but is in an excited state. This process is called *excitation*.
- The unit of energy in the atomic system is the electron volt (eV),
    - 1 eV = 1.6×10^{-19} joules.

X-ray production

X-rays are produced when energetic (high-speed) electrons bombard a target material and are brought suddenly to rest. This happens inside a small evacuated glass envelope called the *X-ray tube* (see Fig. 2.2).

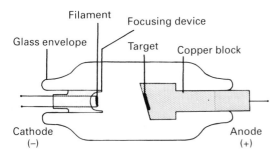

Fig. 2.2 Diagram of a simple X-ray tube showing the main components.

Main features and requirements of an X-ray tube

- The *cathode* (negative) consists of a heated *filament* of tungsten that provides the source of electrons.
- The *anode* (positive) consists of a *target* (a small piece of tungsten) set into the angled face of a large *copper block* to allow efficient removal of heat.
- A *focusing device* aims the stream of electrons at the *focal spot* on the target.
- A high-voltage (kilovoltage, kV) connected between the cathode and anode accelerates the electrons from the negative filament to the positive target. This is sometimes referred to as kVp or kilovoltage peak, as explained later in Chapter 5.
- A current (milliamperage, mA) flows from the cathode to the anode. This is a measure of the quantity of electrons being accelerated.
- A surrounding *lead casing* absorbs unwanted X-rays as a radiation protection measure since X-rays are emitted in all directions.
- Surrounding *oil* facilitates the removal of heat.

Practical considerations

The production of X-rays can be summarized as the following sequence of events:

1. The filament is electrically heated and a cloud of electrons is produced around the filament.
2. The high-voltage (potential difference) across the tube accelerates the electrons at very high speed towards the anode.

3. The focusing device aims the electron stream at the focal spot on the target.
4. The electrons bombard the target and are brought suddenly to rest.
5. The energy lost by the electrons is transferred into either *heat* (about 99%) or X-rays (about 1%).
6. The heat produced is removed and dissipated by the copper block and the surrounding oil.
7. The X-rays are emitted in all directions from the target. Those emitted through the small window in the lead casing constitute the *beam* used for diagnostic purposes.

Interactions at the atomic level

The high-speed electrons bombarding the target (Fig. 2.3) are involved in two main types of *collision* with the tungsten atoms:

- Heat-producing collisions
- X-ray-producing collisions.

Heat-producing collisions

- The incoming electron is deflected by the cloud of outer-shell tungsten electrons, with a small loss of energy, in the form of *heat* (Fig. 2.4A).
- The incoming electron collides with an outer shell tungsten electron displacing it to an even more peripheral shell (excitation) or displacing it from the atom (ionization), again with a small loss of energy in the form of *heat* (Fig. 2.4B).

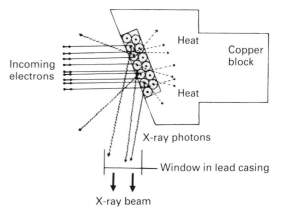

Fig. 2.3 Diagram of the anode enlarged, showing the target and summarizing the interactions at the target.

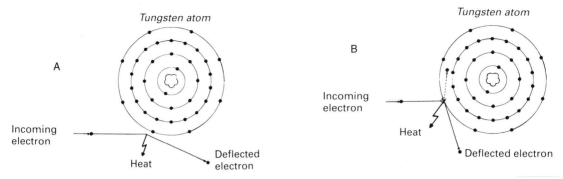

Fig. 2.4A Heat-producing collision: the incoming electron is deflected by the tungsten electron cloud. **B** Heat-producing collision: the incoming electron collides with and displaces an outer-shell tungsten electron.

Important points to note

- Heat-producing interactions are the most common because there are millions of incoming electrons and many outer-shell tungsten electrons with which to interact.
- Each individual bombarding electron can undergo many heat-producing collisions resulting in a considerable amount of heat at the target.
- Heat needs to be removed quickly and efficiently to prevent damage to the target. This is achieved by setting the tungsten target in the copper block, utilizing the high thermal capacity and good conduction properties of copper.

X-ray-producing collisions

- The incoming electron penetrates the outer electron shells and passes close to the nucleus of the tungsten atom. The incoming electron is dramatically slowed down and deflected by the nucleus with a large loss of energy which is emitted in the form of *X-rays* (Fig. 2.5A).
- The incoming electron collides with an inner-shell tungsten electron displacing it to an outer shell (excitation) or displacing it from the atom (ionization), with a large loss of energy and subsequent emission of *X-rays* (Fig. 2.5B).

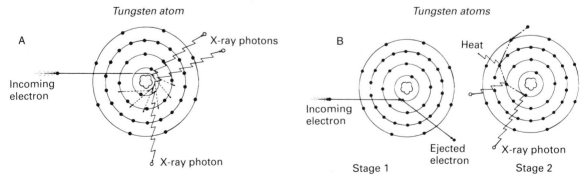

Fig. 2.5A X-ray-producing collision: the incoming electron passes close to the tungsten nucleus and is rapidly slowed down and deflected with the emission of X-ray photons. **B** X-ray-producing collision: Stage 1 — the incoming electron collides with an inner-shell tungsten electron and displaces it; Stage 2 — outer-shell electrons drop into the inner shells with subsequent emission of X-ray photons.

X-ray spectra

The two X-ray-producing collisions result in the production of two different types of *X-ray spectra:*

- Continuous spectrum
- Characteristic spectrum.

Continuous spectrum

The X-ray photons emitted by the rapid deceleration of the bombarding electrons passing close to the nucleus of the tungsten atom are sometimes referred to as *bremsstrahlung* or *braking radiation.* The amount of deceleration and degree of deflection determine the amount of energy lost by the bombarding electron and hence the energy of the resultant emitted photon. A wide range or *spectrum* of photon energies is therefore possible and is termed the *continuous spectrum* (see Fig. 2.6).

Summary of important points

- Small deflections of the bombarding electrons are the most common, producing many *low-energy* photons.

- Low-energy photons have little penetrating power and most will not exit from the X-ray tube itself. They will not contribute to the useful X-ray beam (see Fig. 2.6B). This removal of low-energy photons from the beam is known as *filtration* (see later).
- Large deflections are less likely to happen so there are relatively few *high-energy* photons.
- The maximum photon energy possible (Emax) is directly related to the size of the potential difference (kV) across the X-ray tube.

Characteristic spectrum

Following the ionization or excitation of the tungsten atoms by the bombarding electrons, the orbiting tungsten electrons rearrange themselves to return the atom to the neutral or ground state. This involves electron 'jumps' from one energy level (shell) to another, and results in the emission of X-ray photons with specific energies. As stated previously, the energy levels or shells are specific for any particular atom. The X-ray photons emitted from the target are therefore described as *characteristic of tungsten atoms* and form the *characteristic* or *line spectrum* (see Fig. 2.7). The photon lines are named K and L, depending on the shell from which they have been emitted (see Fig. 2.1).

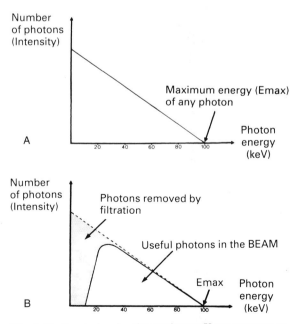

Fig. 2.6A Graph showing the continuous X-ray spectrum at the target for an X-ray tube operating at 100 kV. **B** Graph showing the continuous spectrum in the emitted beam, as the result of *filtration.*

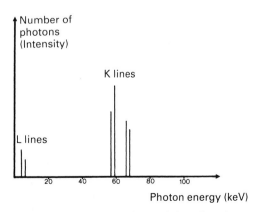

Fig. 2.7 Graph showing the characteristic or line spectrum at the target for an X-ray tube (with a tungsten target) operating at 100 kV.

Summary of important points

- Only the K lines are of diagnostic importance since the L lines have too little energy.
- The bombarding high-speed electron must have sufficient energy (69.5 kV) to displace a K-shell tungsten electron to produce the characteristic K line on the spectrum. (The energy of the bombarding electrons is directly related to the potential difference (kV) across the X-ray tube, see later.)
- Characteristic K-line photons are not produced by X-ray tubes with tungsten targets operating at less than 69.5 kV — referred to as the *critical voltage* (Vc).
- Dental X-ray equipment operates usually between 50 kV and 90 kV (see later).

Combined spectra

In X-ray equipment operating above 69.5 kV, the final total spectrum of the useful X-ray *beam* will be the addition of the continuous and characteristic spectra (see Fig. 2.8).

Summary of the main properties and characteristics of X-rays

- X-rays are *wave packets* of energy of electromagnetic radiation that originate at the atomic level.

- Each *wave packet* is equivalent to a *quantum* of energy and is called a *photon*.
- An X-ray *beam* is made up of millions of photons of different energies.
- The diagnostic X-ray beam can vary in its *intensity* and in its *quality*:
  — Intensity = the number or quantity of X-ray photons in the beam
  — Quality = the energy carried by the X-ray photons which is a measure of their penetrating power.
- The factors that can affect the intensity and/or the quality of the beam include:
  — Size of the tube voltage (kV)
  — Size of the tube current (mA)
  — Distance from the target (d)
  — Time = length of exposure (t)
  — Filtration
  — Target material
  — Tube voltage waveform (see Ch. 5).
- In free space, X-rays travel in straight lines.
- Velocity in free space = 3×10^8 m s^{-1}.
- In free space, X-rays obey the inverse square law:

$$\text{Intensity} = 1/d^2$$

Doubling the distance from an X-ray source reduces the intensity to $\frac{1}{4}$ (a very important principle in radiation protection, see Ch. 6).
- No medium is required for propagation.
- Shorter-wavelength X-rays possess greater energy and can therefore penetrate a greater distance.
- Longer-wavelength X-rays, sometimes referred to as *soft X-rays*, possess less energy and have little penetrating power.
- The energy carried by X-rays can be attenuated by matter, i.e. absorbed or scattered (see later).
- X-rays are capable of producing *ionization* (and subsequent biological damage in living tissue, see Ch. 4) and are thus referred to as *ionizing radiation*.
- X-rays are undetectable by human senses.
- X-rays can affect film emulsion to produce a visual image (the radiograph) and can cause certain salts to fluoresce and to emit light — the principle behind the use of intensifying screens in extraoral cassettes (see Ch. 5).

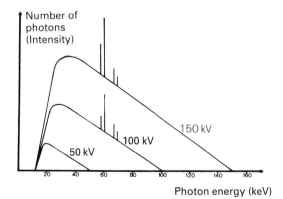

Fig. 2.8 Graphs showing the combination photon energy spectra (in the final beam) for X-ray sets operating at 50 kV, 100 kV and 150 kV.

Interaction of X-rays with matter

When X-rays strike matter, such as a patient's tissues, the photons have four possible fates, shown diagrammatically in Figure 2.9. The photons may be:

- Completely scattered with no loss of energy
- Absorbed with total loss of energy
- Scattered with some absorption and loss of energy
- Transmitted unchanged.

Definition of terms used in X-ray interactions

- *Scattering* — change in direction of a photon with or without a loss of energy
- *Absorption* — deposition of energy, i.e. removal of energy from the beam
- *Attenuation* — reduction in the intensity of the main X-ray beam caused by absorption and scattering

  Attenuation = Absorption + Scattering
- *Ionization* — removal of an electron from a neutral atom producing a negative ion (the electron) and a positive ion (the remaining atom).

Interaction of X-rays at the atomic level

There are four main interactions at the atomic level, depending on the energy of the incoming photon, these include:

- Unmodified or Rayleigh scattering — pure scatter
- Photoelectric effect — pure absorption
- Compton effect — scatter and absorption
- Pair production — pure absorption.

Only two interactions are important in the X-ray energy range used in dentistry:

- Photoelectric effect
- Compton effect.

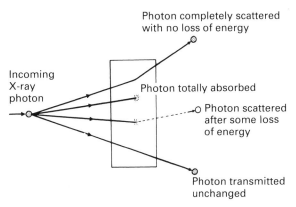

Fig. 2.9 Diagram summarizing the main interactions when X-rays interact with matter.

Photoelectric effect

The photoelectric effect is a pure absorption interaction predominating with *low-energy* photons (see Fig. 2.10).

Summary of the stages in the photoelectric effect

1. The incoming X-ray photon interacts with a bound inner-shell electron of the tissue atom.

2. The inner-shell electron is ejected with considerable energy (now called a *photoelectron*) into the tissues and will undergo further interactions (see below).

3. The X-ray photon disappears having deposited all its energy; the process is therefore one of pure *absorption*.

4. The vacancy which now exists in the inner electron shell is filled by outer-shell electrons dropping from one shell to another.

5. This cascade of electrons to new energy levels results in the emission of excess energy in the form of light or heat.

6. Atomic stability is finally achieved by the capture of a free electron to return the atom to its neutral state.

7. The high-energy ejected *photoelectron* behaves like the original high-energy X-ray photon, undergoing many similar interactions and ejecting other electrons as it passes through the tissues. It is these ejected high-energy electrons that are responsible for the majority of the ionization interactions within tissue, and the possible resulting damage attributable to X-rays.

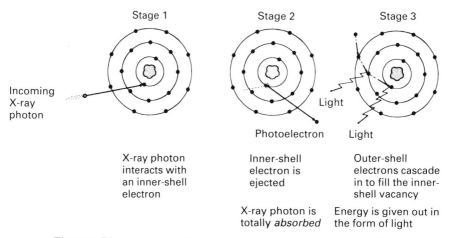

Fig. 2.10 Diagrams representing the stages in the photoelectric interaction.

Important points to note

• The X-ray photon energy needs to be equal to, or just greater than, the binding energy of the inner-shell electron to be able to eject it.

• As the density (atomic number, Z) increases, the number of bound inner-shell electrons also increases. The probability of photoelectric interactions occurring is $\propto Z^3$. Lead has an atomic number of 82 and is therefore a good absorber of X-rays — hence its use in radiation protection (see Ch. 6). The approximate atomic number for soft tissue is 7 ($Z^3 = 343$) and for bone is 12 ($Z^3 = 1728$) — hence their obvious difference in radio-density, and the *contrast* between the different tissues seen on radiographs.

• This interaction predominates with low energy X-ray photons — the probability of photo-electric interactions occurring is $\propto 1/kV^3$. This explains why low kV X-ray equipment results in high absorption (dose) in the patient's tissues, but provides good contrast radiographs.

• The overall result of the interaction is *ionization* of the tissues.

• Intensifying screens, described in Chapter 5, function by the photoelectric effect — when exposed to X-rays, the screens emit their excess energy as *light*, which subsequently affects the film emulsion.

Compton effect

The Compton effect is an absorption *and* scattering process predominating with *higher-energy* photons (see Fig. 2.11).

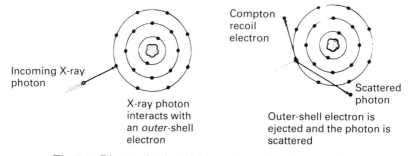

Fig. 2.11 Diagram showing the interactions of the Compton effect.

Summary of the stages in the Compton effect

1. The incoming X-ray photon interacts with a *free* or loosely bound outer-shell electron of the tissue atom.

2. The outer-shell electron is ejected (now called the *Compton recoil electron*) with some of the energy of the incoming photon, i.e. there is some *absorption*. The ejected electron then undergoes further ionizing interactions within the tissues (as before).

3. The remainder of the incoming photon energy is deflected or *scattered* from its original path as a scattered photon.

4. The scattered photon may then:
   - Undergo further Compton interactions within the tissues
   - Undergo photoelectric interactions within the tissues
   - Escape from the tissues — it is these photons that form the *scatter radiation* of concern in the clinical environment.

5. Atomic stability is again achieved by the capture of another free electron.

Important points to note

- The energy of the incoming X-ray photon is much greater than the binding energy of the outer-shell or free electron.

- The incoming X-ray photon cannot distinguish between one free electron and another — the interaction is not dependent on the atomic number (Z). Thus, this interaction provides very little diagnostic information as there is very little discrimination between different tissues on the final radiograph.

- This interaction predominates with high X-ray photon energies. This explains why high-voltage X-ray sets result in radiographs with poor contrast.

- The energy of the scattered photon (Es) is always less than the energy of the incoming photon (E), depending on the energy given to the recoil electron (e):

$$Es = E - e$$

- Scattered photons can be deflected in any direction, but the angle of scatter (θ) depends on their energy. *High-energy* scattered photons produce *forward* scatter; *low-energy* scattered photons produce *back* scatter (see Fig. 2.12).

- Forward scatter may reach the film and degrade the image, but can be removed by using an *anti-scatter grid*.

- The overall result of the interaction is ionization of the tissues.

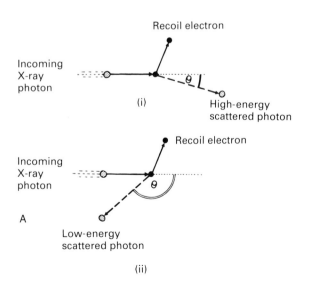

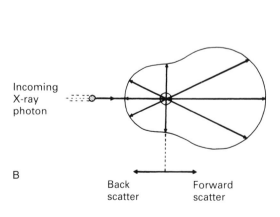

Fig. 2.12A Diagram showing the angle of scatter θ with (i) high - and (ii) low-energy scattered photons. **B** Typical scatter distribution diagram of a 70 kV X-ray set. The length of any radius from the source of scatter indicates the relative amount of scatter in that direction. At this voltage, the majority of scatter is in a forward direction.

3 Dose units and dosimetry

Several different terms and units have been used in dosimetry over the years. The recent conversion to SI units has made this subject even more confusing. However, it is essential that these terms and units are understood to appreciate what is meant by *radiation dose* and to allow meaningful comparisons between different investigations to be made. In addition to explaining the various units, this chapter also summarizes the various sources of ionizing radiation and the magnitude of *radiation doses* that are encountered.

The more important terms in dosimetry include:

- Radiation-absorbed dose (D)
- Equivalent dose (H)
- Effective dose (E)
- Collective effective dose or Collective dose
- Dose rate.

Radiation-absorbed dose (D)

This is a measure of the amount of energy absorbed from the radiation beam per unit mass of tissue.

SI unit : Gray, (Gy) measured in
joules/kg
subunit : milligray, (mGy) ($\times 10^{-3}$)
original unit : rad, measured in ergs/g
conversion : 1 Gray = 100 rads

Equivalent dose (H)

This is a measure which allows the different radiobiological effectiveness (RBE) of different types of radiation to be taken into account.

For example, alpha particles (see Ch. 17) penetrate only a few millimetres in tissue, lose all their energy and are totally absorbed, whereas X-rays penetrate much further, lose some of their energy and are only partially absorbed. The biological effect of a particular *radiation-absorbed dose* of alpha particles would therefore be considerably more severe than a similar *radiation-absorbed dose* of X-rays.

By introducing a numerical value known as the *radiation weighting factor* W_R which represents the biological effects of different radiations, the unit of *equivalent dose (H)* provides a common unit allowing comparisons to be made between one type of radiation and another, for example:

X-rays, gamma rays and beta particles $W_R = 1$
Fast neutrons (10 keV–100 keV)
and protons $W_R = 10$
Alpha particles $W_R = 20$

Equivalent dose (H) = radiation-absorbed dose (D) × radiation weighting factor (W_R)

SI unit : Sievert (Sv)
subunits : millisievert (mSv) ($\times 10^{-3}$)
microsievert (μSv) ($\times 10^{-6}$)
original unit : rem
conversion : 1 Sievert = 100 rems

(For X-rays, the radiation weighting factor (W_R factor) = 1, therefore the *equivalent dose (H)*, measured in *Sieverts*, is equal to the *radiation-absorbed dose (D)*, measured in *Grays*.)

Effective dose (E)

This measure allows doses from different investigations of different parts of the body to be compared, by converting all doses to an *equivalent whole body dose*.

This is necessary because some parts of the body are more sensitive to radiation than others. The International Commission on Radiological Protection (ICRP) has allocated each tissue a numerical value, known as the *tissue weighting factor (W$_T$)*, based on its radiosensitivity, i.e. the risk of the tissue being damaged by radiation — the greater the risk, the higher the *tissue weighting factor*. The sum of the individual *tissue weighting factors* represents the *weighting factor* for the whole body. The *tissue weighting factors* recommended by the ICRP are shown in Table 3.1.

Effective dose (E) = **equivalent dose (H)** × **tissue weighting factor (W$_T$)**

SI unit : Sievert (Sv)
subunit : millisievert (mSv)

When the simple term *dose* is applied loosely, it is the *effective dose (E)* that is usually being described. *Effective dose* can thus be thought of as a broad indication of the risk to health from any exposure to ionizing radiation, irrespective of the type or energy of the radiation or the part of the body being irradiated. A comparison of effective doses from different investigations is shown in Table 3.3.

Collective effective dose or collective dose

This measure is used when considering the total *effective dose* to a *population*, from a particular investigation or source of radiation.

Collective dose = **effective dose (E)** × **population**

SI unit : man-sievert (man-Sv)

Dose rate

This is a measure of the dose per unit time, e.g. dose/hour, and is sometimes a more convenient, and measurable, figure than, for example, a total annual dose limit (see Ch. 6).

SI unit : microsievert/hour (μSv h^{-1})

Table 3.1 The tissue weighting factors (W$_T$) recommended by the ICRP

Tissue	Weighting factor
Gonads	0.2
Red bone marrow	0.12
Colon	0.12
Lung	0.12
Stomach	0.12
Bladder	0.05
Breast	0.05
Liver	0.05
Oesophagus	0.05
Thyroid	0.05
Skin	0.01
Bone surface	0.01
Remainder	0.05

Estimated annual doses from various sources of radiation

Everyone is exposed to some form of ionizing radiation from the environment in which we live. Sources include:

- Natural background radiation
  — Cosmic radiation from the earth's atmosphere
  — Gamma radiation from the rocks and soil in the earth's crust
  — Radiation from ingested radioisotopes, e.g. ^{40}K, in certain foods
  — Radon and its decay products, ^{222}Rn is a gaseous decay product of uranium that is present naturally in granite. As a gas, radon diffuses readily from rocks through soil and can be trapped in poorly ventilated houses and then breathed into the lungs. In the UK, this is of particular concern in areas of Cornwall and Scotland where houses have been built on large deposits of granite
- Artificial background radiation
  — Fallout from nuclear explosions
  — Radioactive waste discharged from nuclear establishments
- Medical and dental diagnostic radiation
- Radiation from occupational exposure.

The National Radiological Protection Board (NRPB) have estimated the annual doses from these various sources in the UK. Table 3.2. gives a summary of the data.

Table 3.2 NRPB-estimated average annual doses to the UK population from various sources of radiation

Radiation source	Average annual dose (μSv)	Approximate %
Natural background		
Cosmic rays	300	
External exposure from the earth's crust	400	
Internal radiation from certain foodstuffs	370	
Exposure to radon and its decay products	700	
Total	2 mSv (approx.)	87%
Artificial background		
Fallout	10	
Radioactive waste	2	>1%
Medical and dental diagnostic radiation	250	12%
Occupational exposure	9	>1%

Table 3.3 Typical effective doses to standard adult patients for a range of dental and routine medical diagnostic examinations

X-ray examination	Effective dose (mSv)
CT chest	8.0
CT head	2.0
Barium swallow	1.5
Barium enema	7.0
Lumbar spine (AP)	0.7
Skull (PA)	0.03
Skull (Lat)	0.01
Chest (PA)	0.02
Chest (Lat)	0.04
Dental panoramic tomograph	
— excluding the salivary glands	0.007–0.014
— including the salivary glands	0.016–0.026
2 dental intraoral films	
— using 70 kV, 200 mm fsd, rectangular collimation and E speed film	0.002
— using 50 kV, 100 mm fsd, round collimation and D speed film	0.016

An individual's average dose from background radiation is estimated at approximately **2 mSv per year** in the UK, while in the USA it is estimated at approximately **3.6 mSv**. These figures are useful to remember when considering the magnitude of the doses associated with various diagnostic procedures (see later).

Typical doses encountered in diagnostic radiology

The NRPB and the Royal College of Radiologists' document *Guidelines on Radiological Standards for Primary Dental Care*, published in 1994, provides examples of typical effective doses for a range of dental examinations using different equipment and image receptors. These are shown in Table 3.3 together with a selection of typical effective doses from various medical diagnostic procedures published in the NRPB document *Guidelines on Patient Dose to Promote the Optimisation of Protection for Diagnostic Medical Exposures* in 1999.

It must be stressed that these are typical values and that a considerable range of effective doses exists in dental radiography. The main reasons for this variation are kV of equipment used, shape and size of beam, speed of film used and the tissues included in the calculations. These factors are of great importance in radiation protection and are discussed in more detail in Chapters 5 and 6.

However, the figures do provide an indication of the comparative sizes of the various effective doses. The individual doses encountered in dental radiology may appear very small, but it must be remembered that the diagnostic burden, however small, is an additional radiation burden to that which the patient is already receiving from background radiation. This additional dose may be considerable for any individual patient. The enormous number of dental radiographs (intraoral and extraoral) taken per year (estimated at approximately 20-25 million in the UK alone) means that the ***collective dose*** from dental radiography is quite substantial. The risks associated with some of the diagnostic investigations are discussed in Chapter 4.

4 The biological effects and risks associated with X-rays

Classification of the biological effects

The biologically damaging effects of ionizing radiation are classified into three main categories:

- Somatic DETERMINISTIC effects
- Somatic STOCHASTIC effects
- Genetic STOCHASTIC effects.

The somatic effects are further subdivided into:

- *Acute* or *immediate* effects — appearing shortly after exposure, e.g. as a result of large whole body doses (Table 4.1)
- *Chronic* or *long-term* effects — becoming evident after a long period of time, the so-called *latent period* (20 years or more), e.g. leukaemia.

Table 4.1 Summary of the main *acute effects* following large whole-body doses of radiation

Dose	Whole-body effect
0.25 Sv	Nil
0.25–1.0 Sv	Slight blood changes, e.g. decrease in white blood cell count
1–2 Sv	Vomiting in 3 hours, fatigue, loss of appetite, blood changes Recovery in a few weeks
2–6 Sv	Vomiting in 2 hours, severe blood changes, loss of hair within 2 weeks Recovery in 1 month to 1 year for 70%
6–10 Sv	Vomiting in 1 hour, intestinal damage, severe blood changes Death in 2 weeks for 80–100%
>10 Sv	Brain damage, coma, death

Somatic deterministic effects

These are the damaging effects to the body of the person exposed that will **definitely** result from a specific high dose of radiation. Examples include skin reddening and cataract formation. The severity of the effect is proportional to the dose received, and in most cases a *threshold* dose exists below which there will be no effect.

Somatic stochastic effects

Stochastic effects are those that **may** develop. Their development is random and depends on the laws of chance or probability. Examples of somatic stochastic effects include leukaemia and certain tumours.

These damaging effects **may** be induced when the body is exposed to **any** dose of radiation. Experimentally it has not been possible to establish a *safe dose* — i.e. a dose below which stochastic effects do not develop. It is therefore assumed that there is *no threshold dose*, and that every exposure to ionizing radiation carries with it the **possibility** of inducing a stochastic effect.

The lower the radiation dose, the lower the probability of cell damage. However, the severity of the damage is **not related** to the size of the inducing dose. This is the underlying philosophy behind present radiation protection recommendations (see Ch. 6).

Genetic stochastic effects

Mutations result from any sudden change to a gene or chromosome. They can be caused by external factors, such as radiation or may occur spontaneously.

Radiation to the reproductive organs **may** damage the DNA of the sperm or egg cells. This **may** result in a congenital abnormality in the off-spring of the person irradiated. However, there is no certainty that these effects will happen, so all genetic effects are described as stochastic.

A cause-and-effect relationship is difficult, if not impossible, to prove. Although ionizing radiation has the potential to cause genetic damage, there are no human data that show convincing evidence of a direct link with radiation. Risk estimates have been based mainly on experiments with mice. It is estimated that a dose to the gonads of 0.5–1.0 Sv would double the spontaneous mutation rate. Once again it is assumed that there is *no threshold dose*.

Effects on the unborn child

The developing fetus is particularly sensitive to the effects of radiation, especially during the period of organogenesis (2–9 weeks after conception). The major problems are:

- Congenital abnormalities or death associated with large doses of radiation
- Mental retardation associated with low doses of radiation.

As a result, the maximum permissible dose to the abdomen of a woman who is pregnant is regulated by law. This is discussed further in Chapter 6.

Harmful effects important in dental radiology

In dentistry, the size of the doses used routinely are relatively small (see Ch. 3) and well below the threshold doses required to produce the somatic deterministic effects. However, the somatic and genetic stochastic effects can develop with **any** dose of ionizing radiation. Dental radiology does not usually involve irradiating the reproductive organs, thus in dentistry somatic stochastic effects are the damaging effects of most concern.

How do X-rays cause damage?

The precise mechanism of how X-rays cause these damaging effects is not yet fully known, but two main mechanisms are thought to be responsible:

- *Direct damage* to specific targets within the cell
- *Indirect damage* to the cell as a result of the ionization of water or other molecules within the cell.

Direct damage

Specific targets within the cell, probably the chromosomal DNA or RNA in the nucleus, take a *direct hit* from an incoming X-ray photon, or an ejected high-energy electron, which breaks the relatively weak bonds between the nucleic acids. The subsequent chromosomal effects could include:

- Inability to pass on information
- Abnormal replication
- Cell death
- Only temporary damage — the DNA being repaired successfully before further cell division.

If the radiation hits somatic cells, the effects on the DNA (and hence the chromosomes) could result in a radiation-induced malignancy. If the damage is to reproductive stem cells, the result could be a radiation-induced congenital abnormality.

What actually happens in the cell depends on several factors, including:

- The type and number of nucleic acid bonds that are broken
- The intensity and type of radiation
- The time between exposures
- The ability of the cell to repair the damage
- The stage of the cell's reproductive cycle when irradiated.

Indirect damage

As 75% of each cell consists of water, it is the water molecules that are most likely to be ionized by the incoming X-rays. The effects are shown in Figure 4.1, which illustrates that the damage to the cell results from the *free radicals* produced by the ionization process.

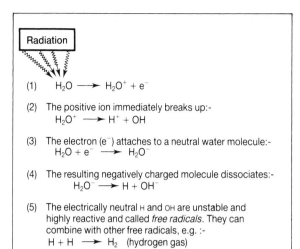

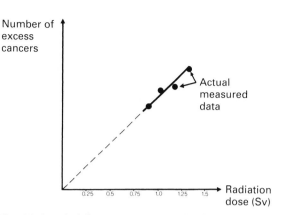

Fig. 4.2 A typical dose–response curve, showing excess cancer incidence plotted against radiation dose and a linear extrapolation of the data to zero.

Fig. 4.1 A diagrammatic summary of the sequence of events following ionization of water molecules leading to *indirect damage* to the cell.

Estimating the magnitude of the risk of cancer induction

Quantifying the risk of somatic stochastic effects, such as radiation-induced cancer, is complex and controversial. Data from groups exposed to **high** doses of radiation are analysed and the results are used to provide an estimate of the risk from the **low** doses of radiation encountered in diagnostic radiology. The high-dose groups studied include:

- The survivors of the atomic explosions at Hiroshima and Nagasaki
- Patients receiving radiotherapy
- Radiation workers — people exposed to radiation in the course of their work
- The survivors of the nuclear disaster at Chernobyl.

The problem of quantifying the risk is compounded because cancer is a common disease, so in any group of individuals studied there is likely to be some incidence of cancer. In the groups listed above, that have been exposed to high doses of radiation, the incidence of cancer is likely to be increased and is referred to as the *excess cancer incidence*. From the data collected, it has been possible

Table 4.2 Broad estimate of the risk of a standard adult patient developing a fatal radiation-induced malignancy from various X-ray examinations (NRPB 1999)

X-ray examination	Estimated risk of fatal cancer
Dental intraoral (× 2)	1 in 2 000 000
Dental panoramic tomograph	1 in 2 000 000
Skull (PA)	1 in 670 000
Skull (Lat)	1 in 2 000 000
Chest (PA)	1 in 1 000 000
Lumbar spine (AP)	1 in 29 000
Barium swallow	1 in 13 000
Barium enema	1 in 3 000
CT chest	1 in 2 500
CT head	1 in 10 000

to construct *dose–response curves* (Fig. 4.2), showing the relationship between excess cancers and radiation dose. The graphs can be extrapolated to zero (the controversy on risk assessment revolves around exactly **how** this extrapolation should be done), and a *risk factor* for induction of cancer by low doses of radiation can be calculated.

A broad estimate of the magnitude of the risk of developing a fatal radiation-induced cancer, from various X-ray examinations, was published in the UK in 1999 by the NRPB in their booklet *Guidelines on Patient Dose to Promote the Optimisation of Protection for Diagnostic Medical Exposures*. These are shown in Table 4.2. *The effective doses (E)* for these examinations were shown in Table 3.3 (p. **27**).

The figures in Table 4.2 show the estimated lifetime risk for patients aged 16–69. Risk is age-dependent, being highest for the young and lowest for the elderly. The NRPB suggests that for children the risk estimates should be multiplied by two and for geriatric patients to be divided by five.

This epidemiological information is being updated continually and recent reports suggest that the risk from low-dose radiation may be considerably greater than thought previously. However, the present figures at least provide an idea of the comparative order of magnitude of the risk involved from different investigations. This in turn helps keep the risks associated with dental radiology in perspective.

Summary

The biological effects of ionizing radiation can be extremely damaging. *Somatic deterministic effects* predominate with **high** doses of radiation, while *somatic stochastic effects* predominate with **low** doses. Dental radiology employs low doses and the risk of stochastic effects is very small. The estimated risk of a fatal cancer developing from two average intraoral bitewing exposures is of the order of one tumour for every 2 million exposures.

In view of the fact that it is estimated that 20 million intraoral and extraoral dental radiographs are taken per year in the UK, it can readily be estimated that the overall risk from dental radiography in this country to be in the order of 10 fatal malignancies per year. The various important dose-reduction and dose-limitation measures that are therefore necessary to keep all exposures *as low as reasonably practicable* (ALARP), for both patients and for dental staff, are outlined in Chapter 6.

5 X-ray equipment, films and processing

This chapter summarizes the more important points of the equipment and the other practical aspects involved in the production of the final radiographic image, namely:

- X-ray generating equipment — required to produce the X-rays
- Image receptors (usually radiographic film) — required to detect the X-rays
- Processing facilities — required to produce the visual black, white and grey image.

Dental X-ray generating equipment

There are several dental X-ray sets available from different manufacturers. They are essentially very similar and can be either *fixed* (wall-mounted or ceiling-mounted) or *mobile* (see Fig. 5.1). They all consist of three main components:

- A tubehead
- Positioning arms
- A control panel and circuitry.

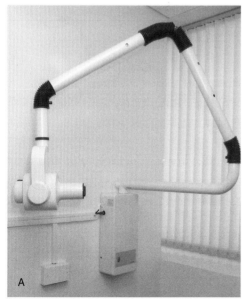
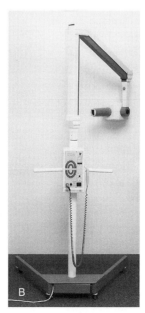
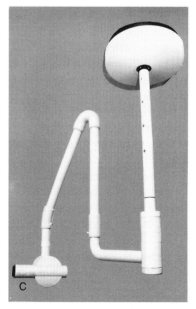

Fig. 5.1 Various styles of dental X-ray sets. **A** Wall-mounted. **B** Mobile. **C** Ceiling-mounted.

Ideal requirements

The equipment should be:

- Safe and accurate
- Capable of generating X-rays in the desired energy range and with adequate mechanisms for heat removal
- Small
- Easy to manoeuvre and position
- Stable, balanced and steady once the tubehead has been positioned
- Easily folded and stored
- Simple to operate
- Robust.

Main components of the tubehead

A diagram of a typical tubehead is shown in Figure 5.2. The main components include:

- The *glass X-ray tube*, including the filament, copper block and the target (see Ch. 2)
- The *step-up transformer* required to step-up the mains voltage of 240 volts to the high voltage (kV) required across the X-ray tube
- The *step-down transformer* required to step-down the mains voltage of 240 volts to the low voltage current required to heat the filament
- A *surrounding lead shield* to minimize leakage
- *Surrounding oil* to facilitate heat removal
- *Aluminium filtration* to remove harmful low-energy (soft) X-rays
- The *collimator* — a metal disc or cylinder with central aperture designed to shape and limit the beam size to a rectangle (the same size as intraoral film) or round with a maximum diameter of 6 cm
- The *spacer cone* or *beam-indicating device (BID)* — a device for indicating the direction of the beam and setting the ideal distance from the focal spot on the target to the skin. The legal focus to skin (fsd) distances are:
  — 200 mm for sets operating above 60 kV
  — 100 mm for sets operating below 60 kV
  There are several designs of spacer cone available, varying in shape, material and length, as well as adaptors to change the shape of the emerging X-ray beam (see Fig. 5.3 and Fig. 5.4).

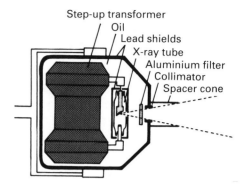

Fig. 5.2 Diagram of the tubehead of a typical dental X-ray set showing the main components.

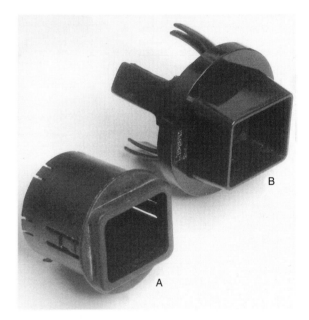

Fig. 5.3 Examples of adaptors/collimators designed to change the shape of the beam from circular to rectangular. **A** Siemens Heliodent collimator, **B** Dentsply's Universal collimator.

Focal spot size and the principle of line focus

As stated in Chapter 1, the focal spot (the source of the X-rays) should be ideally a *point source* to reduce blurring of the image — the *penumbra effect* — as shown in Figure 5.5A. However, the heat produced at the target by the bombarding electrons needs to be distributed over as large an area as possible. These two opposite requirements are satisfied by using an angled target and the principle of *line focus*, as shown in Figure 5.5B.

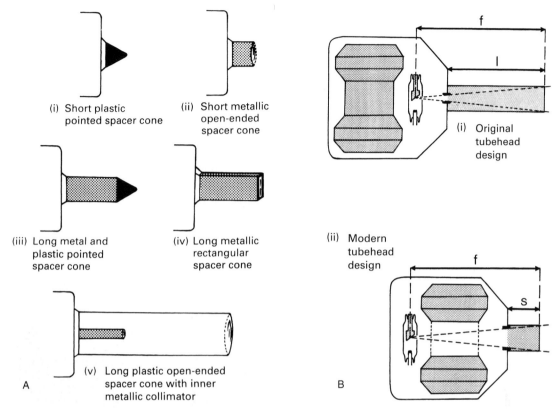

Fig. 5.4A Diagrams showing various designs and shapes of spacer cones or beam-indicating devices. **Note:** The short plastic pointed spacer cone is NOT recommended. **B** Diagrams showing (i) the original tubehead design with the X-ray tube at the **front** of the head, thus requiring a long spacer cone (1) to achieve a parallel X-ray beam and the correct focus to skin distance (f) and (ii) the modern tubehead design with the X-ray tube at the **back** of the head, thus requiring only a short spacer cone (s) to achieve the same focus to skin distance (f).

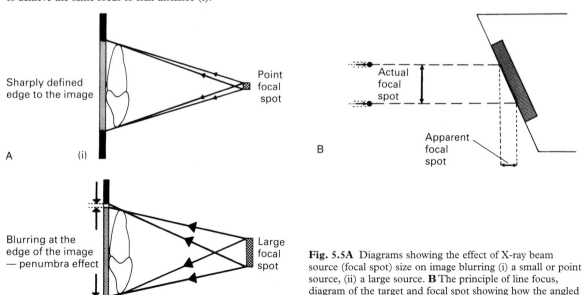

Fig. 5.5A Diagrams showing the effect of X-ray beam source (focal spot) size on image blurring (i) a small or point source, (ii) a large source. **B** The principle of line focus, diagram of the target and focal spot showing how the angled target face allows a large *actual* focal spot but a small *apparent* focal spot.

Main components of the control panel

Examples of two typical control panels are shown in Figure 5.6. The main components include:

- The *mains on/off* switch and *warning light*
- The *timer*, of which there are three main types:
  — electronic
  — impulse
  — clockwork (inaccurate and no longer used)
- An *exposure time selector* mechanism, usually either:
  — numerical, time selected in seconds
  — anatomical, area of mouth selected and exposure time adjusted automatically
- *Warning lights* and *audible signals* to indicate when X-rays are being generated
- Other features can include:
  — *Film speed selector*
  — *Patient size selector*
  — *Mains voltage compensator*
  — *Kilovoltage selector*
  — *Milliamperage switch*
  — *Exposure adjustment for long or short fsd.*

Circuitry and tube voltage

The mains supply to the X-ray machine of 240 volts has two functions:

- To generate the high potential difference (kV) to accelerate the electrons across the X-ray tube via the step-up transformer
- To provide the low-voltage current to heat the tube filament via the step-down transformer.

However, the incoming 240 volts is an alternating current with the typical waveform shown in Figure 5.7. Half the cycle is positive and the other half is negative. For X-ray production, only the positive half of the cycle can be used to ensure that the electrons from the filament are always drawn towards the target. Thus, the stepped-up high voltage applied across the X-ray tube needs to be *rectified* to eliminate the negative half of the cycle. Four types of rectified circuits are used:

- Half-wave rectified
- Single-phase, full-wave rectified
- Three-phase, full-wave rectified
- Constant potential.

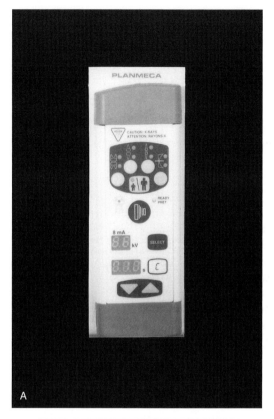

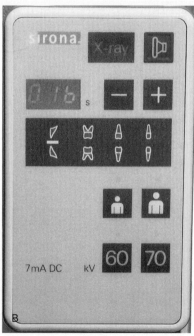

Fig. 5.6 Control panel of **A** Planmeca Prostyle and **B** Siemens (Sirona) Heliodent.

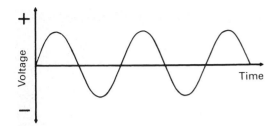

Fig. 5.7 Diagram showing the alternating current waveform.

The waveforms resulting from these rectified circuits, together with graphical representation of their subsequent X-ray production, are shown in Figure 5.8. These changing waveforms mean that equipment is only working at its optimum or peak output at the top of each cycle. The kilovoltage is therefore often described as the *kVpeak* or *kVp*. Thus a 50 kVp half-wave rectified X-ray set only in fact functions at 50 kV for a tiny fraction of the time of any exposure.

Modern designs favour constant potential circuity, often referred to as *DC units*, which keep the kilovoltage at kVpeak throughout any exposure, thus ensuring that:

- X-ray production per unit time is more efficient
- More high-energy, diagnostically useful photons are produced per exposure
- Fewer low energy, harmful photons are produced
- Shorter exposure times are possible.

Other X-ray generating apparatus

The other common X-ray generating equipment encountered in dentistry includes:

- Panoramic X-ray machines
- Skull units, such as the Craniotome® or Orbix®
- Cephalometric skull equipment.

The main features and practical components of relevant machines are outlined in later chapters.

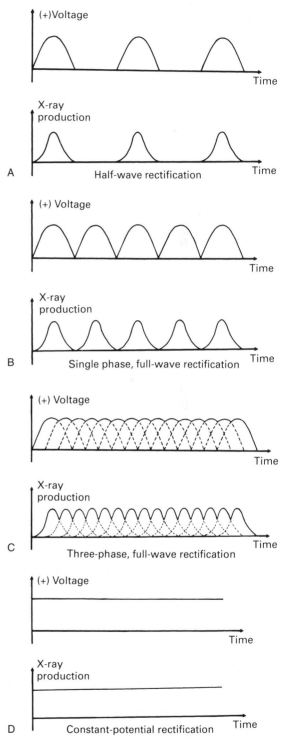

Fig. 5.8 Diagrams showing the waveforms and X-ray production graphs resulting from different forms of rectification.

Image receptors

The usual image receptor used in dentistry is radiographic film. There are two basic types:

- *Direct-action* or *non-screen* film (sometimes referred to as *wrapped* or *packet* film). This type of film is sensitive primarily to X-ray photons.
- *Indirect-action* or *screen* film, so-called because it is used in combination with *intensifying screens* in a *cassette*. This type of film is sensitive primarily to light photons, which are emitted by the adjacent intensifying screens.

The advantage of intensifying screens and indirect-action film is that they respond to a shorter exposure of X-rays, enabling a lower dose of radiation to be given to the patient. However, this is at the cost of inferior image quality.

A summary of the main features of both types of image detector is given below.

Direct-action (non-screen) film

Uses

Direct-action film is used for intraoral radiography where the need for excellent image quality and fine anatomical detail are of importance.

Sizes

Various sizes of film are available, although only three are usually used routinely (see Fig. 5.9).

- 31 × 41 mm — for periapicals and
- 22 × 35 mm — bitewings
- 57 × 76 mm — for occlusals.

The film packet contents

The contents of a film packet are shown in Figure 5.10.

Important points to note

- The outer packet or wrapper is made of non-absorbent paper or plastic and is sealed to prevent the ingress of saliva.
- The side of the packet that faces towards the X-ray beam has either a pebbled or a smooth surface and is usually white.
- The reverse side is usually of two colours so there is little chance of the film being placed the wrong way round in the patient's mouth and different colours represent different film speeds.
- The black paper on either side of the film is there to protect the film from:
  - Light
  - Damage by fingers while being unwrapped
  - Saliva which may leak into the film packet.
- A thin sheet of lead foil is placed behind the film to prevent:
  - Some of the residual radiation that has passed through the film from continuing on into the patient's tissues
  - Scattered secondary radiation, from X-ray photon interactions within the tissues

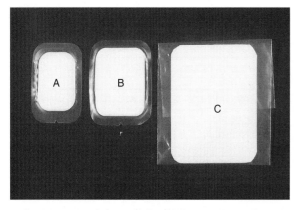

Fig. 5.9 The typical sizes of barrier-wrapped direct-action radiographic film packets available. **A** Small periapical/ bitewing film. **B** Large periapical/bitewing film. **C** Occlusal film.

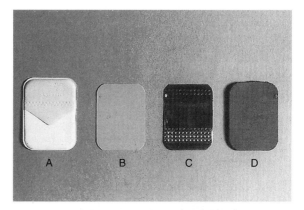

Fig. 5.10 The contents of a film packet. **A** The outer wrapper. **B** The film. **C** The sheet of lead foil. **D** The protective black paper.

beyond the film, coming back on to the film and degrading the image.

• The sheet of lead foil contains an embossed pattern so that should the film packet be placed the wrong way round, the pattern will appear on the resultant radiograph. This enables the cause of the resultant underexposed pale film to be easily identified (see Ch. 16).

The radiographic film

The cross-sectional structure and components of the radiographic film are shown in Figure 5.11.

The radiographic film comprises four basic components:

• A *plastic base*, made of clear, transparent cellulose acetate which acts as a support for the emulsion but does not contribute to the final image

• A thin layer of *adhesive* that fixes the emulsion to the base

• The *emulsion* on **both** sides of the base — this consists of silver halide (usually bromide) crystals embedded in a gelatin matrix. The X-ray photons *sensitize* the silver halide crystals that they strike and these sensitized silver halide crystals are later reduced to visible black metallic silver in the developer (see later)

• A *protective layer* of clear gelatin to shield the emulsion from mechanical damage.

Film orientation

The film has an embossed *dot* on one corner that is used to help orientation. Its position is marked on the back of the packet or can be felt as a raised dot on the front. The side of the film on which the dot is raised is always placed towards the X-ray beam. When the films are mounted, this raised dot

is towards the operator and the films are then arranged anatomically and viewed as if the operator were facing the patient.

Indirect-action film

Uses

Film/screen combinations are used as image detectors whenever possible because of the reduced dose of radiation to the patient (particularly when very fine image detail is not essential). The main uses include:

• Extraoral projections, including:
— Oblique lateral radiographs (Ch. 11)
— Lateral skull radiographs (Ch. 12)
— Dental panoramic tomographs (Ch. 13)
— All routine medical radiography
• The intraoral, vertex occlusal radiograph (Ch. 10).

Indirect-action film construction

This type of film is similar in construction to direct-action film described above. However, the following important points should be noted:

• The silver halide emulsion is designed to be sensitive primarily to light rather than X-rays.
• Different emulsions are manufactured which are sensitive to the different colours of light emitted by different types of intensifying screens (see later). These include:
— *Standard silver halide emulsion* sensitive to BLUE light
— *Modified silver halide emulsion with ultraviolet sensitizers* sensitive to ULTRAVIOLET light
— *Orthochromatic emulsion* sensitive to GREEN light
— *Panchromatic emulsion* sensitive to RED light

The relative spectral sensitivity of these four different film emulsions is shown in Figure 5.12.

• It is essential that the correct combination of film and intensifying screens is used.
• There is no orientation *dot* embossed in the film so some form of additional identification is required, e.g. metal letters, **L** or **R** placed on the outside of the cassette or electronic marking.

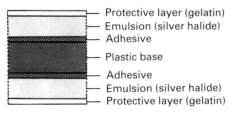

— Protective layer (gelatin)
— Emulsion (silver halide)
— Adhesive
— Plastic base
— Adhesive
— Emulsion (silver halide)
— Protective layer (gelatin)

Fig. 5.11 Diagram showing the cross-sectional structure of double emulsion radiographic film.

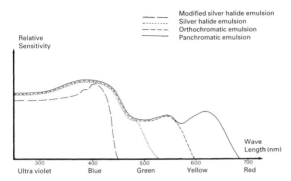

Fig. 5.12 Graph showing the relative spectral sensitivity of standard silver halide (BLUE), modified silver halide (ULTRAVIOLET), orthochromatic (GREEN) and panchromatic (RED) film emulsions.

Characteristics of radiographic film

This section summarizes the more important theoretical terms and definitions used to describe how radiographic film responds to exposure to X-rays.

Optical density (OD)

$$OD = \log \frac{\text{Incident light intensity}}{\text{Transmitted light intensity}}$$

Optical density is the term used for describing the degree of film blackening and can be measured directly using a densitometer. In diagnostic radiology the range of optical densities is usually 0.25–2.5. There are no units for optical density.

Characteristic curve

The characteristic curve is a graph showing the variation in optical density (degree of blackening) with different exposures. Typical characteristic curves for direct-action (non-screen) and indirect-action (screen) film are shown in Figure 5.13. This curve describes several of the film's properties.

Background fog density

This is the small degree of blackening evident even with zero exposure. This is due to:

- The colour/density of the plastic base
- The development of some unexposed silver halide crystals.

If the film has been stored correctly (see later), this background fog density should be less than 0.2 (see Fig. 5.13).

Film speed

This is the exposure required to produce an optical density of 1.0 above background fog (see Fig. 5.14). Thus, the faster the film, the less the exposure required for a given film blackening and the lower the radiation dose to the patient.

Film speed is a function of the number and size of the silver halide crystals in the emulsion. The larger the crystals, the faster the film but the poorer the image quality.

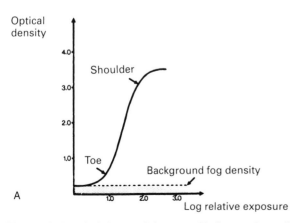

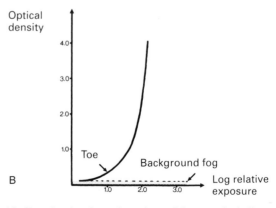

Fig. 5.13A A typical characteristic curve of indirect-action radiographic film, showing the main regions of the curve including *background fog density*, *toe* and *shoulder*. **B** A typical characteristic curve for direct-action film.

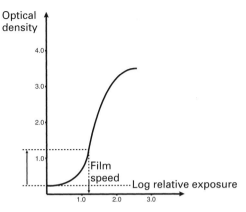

Fig. 5.14 The characteristic curve of an indirect-action (screen) film showing the *film speed* — the exposure required to produce an optical density of 1.0 above background fog.

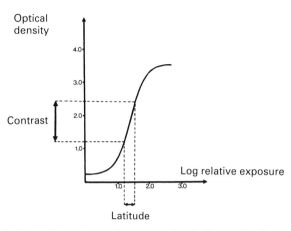

Fig. 5.15 The characteristic curve of an indirect-action film showing film *contrast* and *latitude*.

In clinical practice, the fastest films consistent with adequate diagnostic results, either D speed or more usually nowadays the faster E or F speed, should be used.

Film sensitivity

This is the reciprocal of the exposure required to produce an optical density of 1.0 above background fog. Thus, a fast film has a high sensitivity.

Film latitude

This is a measure of the range of exposures that produces distinguishable differences in optical density, i.e. the linear portion of the characteristic curve (see Fig. 5.15). The wider the film latitude the greater the range of object densities that may be seen.

Film contrast

This is the difference in optical density between two points on a film that have received different exposures (see Fig. 5.15).

Film gamma and average gradient

Film gamma is the *maximum* gradient or slope of the linear portion of the characteristic curve. This term is often quoted but is of little value in radiology because the maximum slope (steepest)

portion of the characteristic curve is usually very short.

Average gradient is a more useful measurement and is usually calculated between density 0.25 and 2.0 above background fog (see Fig. 5.16).

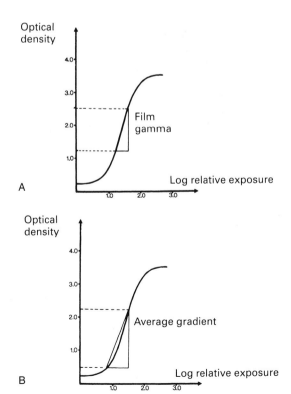

Fig. 5.16 Characteristic curves showing **A** *film gamma* and **B** *average gradient* of an indirect-action (screen) film.

Thus the film *gamma* or *average gradient* measurement determines both *film latitude* and *film contrast* as follows:

- If the gamma or average gradient is **high** (i.e. a steep gradient), that film will show good contrast, but will have less latitude.
- If the film gamma or average gradient is **low** (i.e. a shallow gradient), that film will show poor contrast but will have wider latitude.

Resolution

Resolution, or resolving power, is a measure of the radiograph's ability to differentiate between different structures that are close together. Factors that can affect resolution include penumbra effect (image sharpness), silver halide crystal size and contrast. It is measured in line pairs (lp) per mm. Direct-action film has a resolution of approximately 10 lp per mm and indirect-action film a resolution of about 5 lp per mm.

Intensifying screens

Intensifying screens consist of *fluorescent phosphors*, which emit light when excited by X-rays, embedded in a plastic matrix. The basic construction and components of an intensifying screen are shown in Figure 5.17.

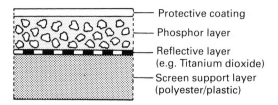

Fig. 5.17 Diagram showing the cross-sectional structure of a typical intensifying screen.

Action

Two intensifying screens are used — one in front of the film and the other at the back. The front screen absorbs the low-energy X-ray photons and the back screen absorbs the high-energy photons. The two screens are therefore efficient at stopping the transmitted X-ray beam, which they convert into visible light by the *photoelectric effect* (described in Ch. 2). One X-ray photon will produce many light photons which will affect a relatively large area of film emulsion. Thus, the amount of radiation needed to expose the film is reduced but at the cost of fine detail; *resolution* is decreased. The ultraviolet system has been developed recently to improve *resolution* by reducing light diffusion and having virtually no light crossover through the plastic film base (see Fig. 5.18).

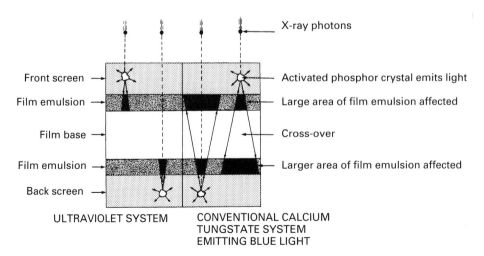

Fig. 5.18 Diagram showing the action of conventional calcium tungstate and ultraviolet systems. Note the small cone of ultraviolet light with no crossover through the film base, compared to the large cone of blue light and marked crossover from the calcium tungstate phosphors. These differences result in better resolution and image sharpness with ultraviolet systems.

Useful definitions

The following terms are used to describe intensifying screens:

- *Conversion efficiency* — the efficiency with which the phosphor converts X-rays into light
- *Absorption efficiency* — the ability of the phosphor material to absorb X-rays
- *Screen efficiency* — the ability of the light emitted by the phosphor to escape from the screen and expose the film
- *Intensification factor* (IF)

$$IF = \frac{\text{Exposure required when screens are not used}}{\text{Exposure required with screens}}$$

- *Screen speed* — the time taken for the screen to emit light following exposure to X-rays. The faster the screen, the lower the radiation dose to the patient.
- *Packing density* — the ability of the phosphor to pack closely together resulting in thin screens and less light divergence.

Fluorescent materials

Three main phosphor materials are used in intensifying screens:

- Calcium tungstate ($CaWO_4$)
- Rare earth phosphors including gadolinium and lanthanum
- Yttrium (a non-rare earth phosphor but having similar properties).

Calcium tungstate screens

The main points can be summarized as follows:

- The speed of these screens depends upon:
  - The thickness of the phosphor layer
  - The size of the phosphor crystals
  - The presence or absence of light-absorbing dyes within the screen
  - The *conversion efficiency* of the crystals
- The faster the screen, the lower the radiation dose to the patient **but** the less the detail of the final image
- **All** calcium tungstate screens emit BLUE light and must be used with blue-light sensitive monochromatic radiographic film (see Fig. 5.19).

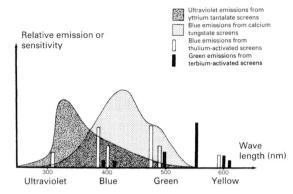

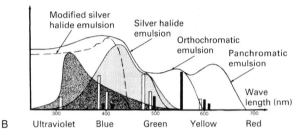

Fig. 5.19A Graph showing the relative spectral emissions of different types of intensifying screens. **B** Graph showing the spectral sensitivity of different types of film combined with the relative spectral emissions of different types of intensifying screens.

Rare earth and related screens

These new phosphors have been introduced to increase screen speeds even more, so further reducing the radiation dose to patients without excessive loss of image detail. The main points can be summarized as follows:

- The rare earth group of elements includes:
  - lanthanum (Z = 57)
  - gadolinium (Z = 64)
  - terbium (Z = 65)
  - thulium (Z = 69)
- The term *rare earth* is used because it is difficult and expensive to separate these elements from earth and from each other, not because the elements are scarce
- These phosphors only fluoresce properly when they contain impurities of other phosphors, e.g. gadolinium plus 0.3% terbium. Typical screens include:

— Terbium-activated gadolinium oxysulphide ($Gd_2O_1S:Tb$)

— Thulium-activated lanthanum oxybromide ($LaOBr:Tm$)

- Terbium-activated screens emit GREEN light, while thulium-activated screens emit BLUE light (see Fig. 5.19)
- Yttrium ($Z = 39$), the rare earth related phosphor, in the form of pure yttrium tantalate ($YTaO_4$) emits ULTRAVIOLET light (see Fig. 5.19)
- Rare earth and related screens are approximately five times faster than calcium tungstate screens. The amount of radiation required to produce an image is therefore considerably reduced, but they are relatively expensive.
- Several different screens of each phosphor, each producing a different *image system speed*, are available:

Screen type	Image system speed
Detail or Fine	100
Fast detail or Medium	200
Rapid or Fast	400
Super rapid	800

- It is important to use the appropriate films with their correctly matched screens.

Cassettes

Types

Cassettes are made in a variety of shapes and sizes for different projections. A selection is shown in Figure 5.20.

Construction

Despite their different shapes, the construction of the cassettes is very similar. They consist usually of a light-tight aluminium or carbon fibre container with the radiographic film sandwiched tightly between two intensifying screens (see Fig. 5.21). Any loss in film/screen contact will result in degradation of the final image.

Important practical points to note

Film storage

All radiographic film deteriorates with time and manufacturers state expiry dates on film boxes as a

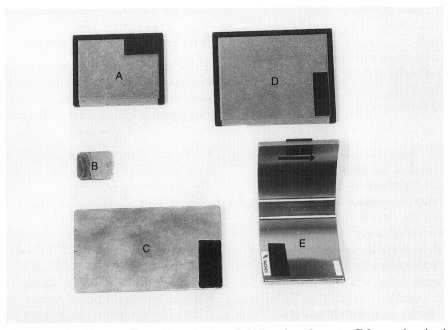

Fig. 5.20 Various cassettes for different radiographic projections. **A** Oblique lateral cassette. **B** Intraoral occlusal cassette. **C** Flat panoramic cassette. **D** Skull cassette. **E** Curved panoramic cassette.

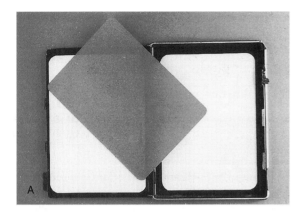

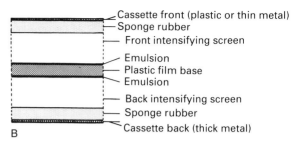

Fig. 5.21A A standard 18 × 13 cm cassette opened up showing the white intensifying screens and the film. **B** Diagram showing the cross-sectional components in a cassette.

guide. However, this does not mean that the film automatically becomes unusable after this date. Storage conditions can have a dramatic effect on the deterioration rate. Ideally films should be stored:

- In a refrigerator in cool, dry conditions
- Away from all sources of ionizing radiation
- Away from chemical fumes including mercury and mercury-containing compounds
- With boxes placed on their edges, to prevent pressure artefacts.

Screen maintenance

Intensifying screens should last for many years if looked after correctly. Maintenance should include:

- Regular cleaning with a proprietary cleaning agent
- Careful handling to avoid scratching or damaging the surface
- Regular checks for loss of film/screen contact.

These aspects are discussed further in Chapter 15.

Processing facilities

Processing is the general term used to describe the sequence of events required to convert the invisible *latent image*, contained in the sensitized film emulsion, into the visible, permanent radiographic image and is usually performed by dental nurses.

It is CRUCIAL that this stage is performed under controlled, standardized conditions with careful attention to detail. Unfortunately, all too often poor processing is the cause of radiographs

being of inadequate diagnostic quality, irrespective of how reliable and expensive the X-ray equipment or how accurate the operator's radiographic techniques.

Processing theory

A detailed knowledge of the chemistry involved in processing is not essential. However, a working knowledge and understanding of the theory of processing is necessary so that processing faults can be identified and corrected. A simplified approach to the stages involved in converting the green film emulsion into the black/white/grey radiograph is shown in Figure 5.22 and outlined below:

Stage 1: Development

The **sensitized** silver halide crystals in the emulsion are converted to black metallic silver to produce the *black/grey* parts of the image.

Stage 2: Washing

The film is washed in water to remove residual developer solution.

Stage 3: Fixation

The **unsensitized** silver halide crystals in the emulsion are removed to reveal the *transparent* or *white* parts of the image and the emulsion is hardened.

Stage 4: Washing

The film is washed thoroughly in running water to remove residual fixer solution.

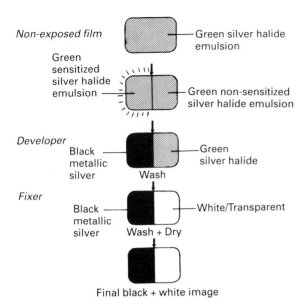

Non-exposed film — Green silver halide emulsion

Green sensitized silver halide emulsion — Green non-sensitized silver halide emulsion

Developer
Black metallic silver — Green silver halide
Wash

Fixer
Black metallic silver — White/Transparent
Wash + Dry

Final black + white image

Fig. 5.22 Diagram showing the stages involved in processing, to convert the green film emulsion to the final black and white radiograph (courtesy of Mrs J.E. Brown).

Stage 5: Drying

The resultant *black/white/grey* radiograph is dried.

Practical processing methods

There are three practical processing methods available:

- Manual or wet processing
- Automatic processing
- Using self-developing films.

Manual processing

Manual processing is usually carried out in a *dark-room*, the general requirements of which should include:

- Absolute light-tightness
- Adequate working space
- Adequate ventilation
- Adequate washing facilities
- Adequate film storage facilities
- Safelights — positioned 1.2 m from the work surfaces with 25 W bulbs and filters suitable for the type of film being used (see Ch 15)
- Processing equipment (see Fig. 5.23):
  — Tanks containing the various solutions
  — Thermometer
  — Immersion heater
  — An accurate timer
  — Film hangers.

Manual processing cycle

1. The exposed film packet is unwrapped and the film clipped on to a hanger.

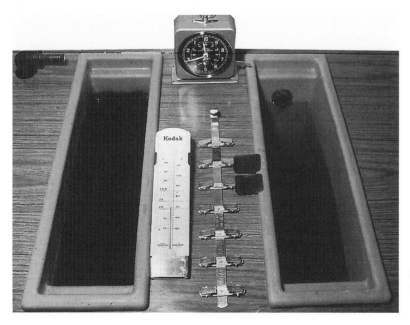

Fig. 5.23 The basic requirements for manual processing including a series of solution tanks, thermometer, timer and film.

2. The film is immersed in DEVELOPER and agitated several times in the solution to remove air bubbles and left for about 5 minutes at 20°C.

3. The residual developer is rinsed off in water for about 10 seconds.

4. The film is immersed in FIXER for about 8–10 minutes.

5. The film is washed in running water for about 10–20 minutes to remove any residual fixer.

6. The film is allowed to dry in a dust-free atmosphere.

Processing solutions

Two different processing solutions are required, the *developer* and the *fixer*. The typical constituents of these solutions are shown in Tables 5.1 and 5.2.

Important points to note regarding development

- The alkaline developer solution should be made up to the concentration recommended in the manufacturer's instructions.

Table 5.1 The typical constituents of developer solution and their functions

Constituents	Functions
Phenidone	Helps bring out the image
Hydroquinone	Builds contrast
Sodium sulphite	Preservative — reduces oxidation
Potassium carbonate	Activator — governs the activity of the developing agents
Benzotriazole	Restrainer — prevents fog and controls the activity of the developing agents
Glutaraldehyde	Hardens the emulsion
Fungicide	Prevents bacterial growth
Buffer	Maintains pH (7+)
Water	Solvent

Table 5.2 The typical constituents of fixer solution and their functions

Constituents	Functions
Ammonium thiosulphate	Removes unsensitized silver halide crystals
Sodium sulphite	Preservative — prevents deterioration of the fixing agent
Aluminium chloride	Hardener
Acetic acid	Acidifier — maintains pH
Water	Solvent

- The developer solution is oxidized by air and its effectiveness decreased. Solutions should be used for no more than 10–14 days, irrespective of the number of films processed during that time.
- If the development process is allowed to continue for too long, more silver will be deposited than was intended and the radiograph will be too dark. Conversely, if there is too short a development time the radiograph will be too light.
- Development TIME (in fresh solutions) is dependent on the TEMPERATURE of the solution. The usual value recommended is 5 minutes at 20°C.
- If the temperature is too high, development is rapid, the film may be too dark and the emulsion may be damaged. If the temperature is too low, development is slowed and a pale film will result.

Important points to note regarding fixing

- Fixer solution should be made up to the concentration recommended by the manufacturer. It is an acid solution so contamination with developer should be avoided.
- Films should ideally be fixed for double the *clearing time*. The clearing time is how long it takes to remove the unsensitized silver halide crystals. Total fixing time is usually 8–10 minutes.
- Films may be removed from the fixer after 2–4 minutes for *wet* viewing but should be returned to the fixer solution to complete fixing.
- Inadequately fixed films may appear greenish yellow or milky owing to residual emulsion. In time these films may discolour further, becoming brown.

Automatic processing

This term is used when processing is carried out automatically by a machine. There are several automatic processors available which are designed to carry the film through the complete cycle usually by a system of rollers. Most have a daylight loading facility, eliminating the need for a darkroom (see Fig. 5.24), but in the interests of infection control, salivary-contaminated film packets should be wiped with a disinfecting solution such as 1% hypochlorite, before being placed into the loading facility.

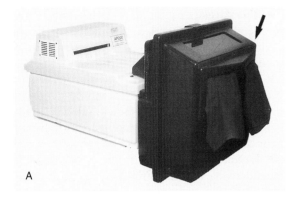

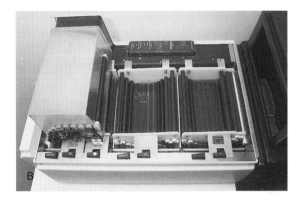

Fig. 5.24A The AP200 automatic processor fitted with its daylight loading apparatus (arrowed). **B** The internal tanks and roller system of the AP200 processor.

Automatic processing cycle

The cycle is the same as for manual processing except that the rollers squeeze off any excess developing solution before passing the film on to the fixer, eliminating the need for the water wash between these two solutions.

Advantages

The main advantages include:

- Time saving — dry films are produced in about 5 minutes
- The need for a darkroom is often eliminated
- Controlled, standardized processing conditions are easy to maintain
- Chemicals can be replenished automatically by some machines.

Disadvantages

The main disadvantages include:

- Strict maintenance and regular cleaning are essential; dirty rollers produce marked films
- Some models need to be plumbed in
- Equipment is relatively expensive
- Smaller machines cannot process large extraoral films.

Self-developing films

Self-developing films are an alternative to manual processing. The X-ray film is presented in a special sachet containing developer and fixer (see Fig. 5.25). Following exposure, the developer tab is

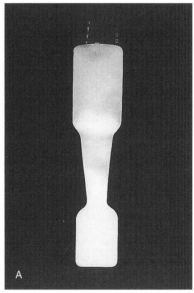

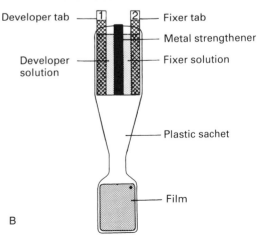

Fig. 5.25A A self-developing film. **B** Diagram showing the basic internal design.

pulled, releasing developer solution which is milked down towards the film and massaged around it. After about 15 seconds, the fixer tab is pulled to release the fixer solution which is similarly milked down to the film. After fixing, the used chemicals are discarded and the film is rinsed thoroughly under running water for about 10 minutes.

Advantages

The main advantages include:

- No darkroom or processing facilities are needed
- Time saving — the final radiograph is ready in about a minute.

Disadvantages

The main disadvantages include:

- Poor overall image quality
- The image deteriorates rapidly with time
- There is no lead foil inside the film packet
- The film packet is very flexible and easily bent
- These films are difficult to use in positioning holders
- Relatively expensive.

A rigid, radiopaque plastic backing support tray for the film is manufactured, which helps to reduce the problems of flexibility and lack of lead foil.

Radiation protection

Part 3

6 Radiation protection

Ionizing radiation is the subject of considerable safety legislation designed to minimize the risks to radiation workers and to patients. The International Commission on Radiological Protection (ICRP) regularly publishes data and general recommendations based on the following general principles:

- No practice shall be adopted unless its introduction produces a positive net benefit (*Justification*)
- All exposures shall be kept **as low as reasonably practicable** (ALARP), taking economic and social factors into account (*Optimization*)
- The dose equivalent to individuals shall not exceed the limits recommended by the ICRP (*Limitation*).

Their recommendations are usually incorporated eventually into national legislation and guidelines, although the precise details may vary from one country to another. By way of illustration, this chapter summarizes the current recommendations, guidelines and legislative requirements in force in the UK, together with the practical radiation protection measures that apply to patients and dental staff.

Current UK legislation and guidelines

Legislation

There are two sets of regulations in the UK governing the use of ionizing radiation. They both form part of The Health and Safety at Work Act 1974 and comply with the provisions of the European Council Directives 96/29/Euratom and 97/43/Euratom:

- ***The Ionising Radiations Regulations 1999 (SI 1999 No. 3232)*** (IRR 99) which replace the Ionising Radiations Regulations 1985 (SI 1985 No. 1333).
- ***The Ionising Radiation (Medical Exposure) Regulations 2000 (SI 2000 No. 1059)*** (IR(ME)R2000) which replace the Ionising Radiation (Protection of Persons Undergoing Medical Examination or Treatment) Regulations 1988 (SI 1988 No. 778).

Guidelines

There are three sets of guidelines, namely:

- *Guidelines on Radiological Standards in Primary Dental Care* published in 1994 by the National Radiological Protection Board (NRPB) and the Royal College of Radiologists. These guidelines and their recommendations cover all aspects of dental radiology and set out the principles of good practice.
- *Selection Criteria for Dental Radiography* first published in 1998 by the Faculty of General Dental Practitioners of the Royal College of Surgeons of England. This booklet reviews the evidence for, and provides guidance on, which radiographs are appropriate for different clinical conditions and how frequently they should be taken. The overview of their recommendations is reproduced later in this chapter.
- *Guidance Notes for Dental Practitioners on the Safe Use of X-ray Equipment* published by the Department of Health in 2001 which brings

together the requirements of IRR99 and IR(ME)R2000 as they relate to dentistry, and includes the principles of good practice established in the 1994 Guidelines. The main points and various extracts from these 2001 *Guidance Notes* are reproduced below with kind permission from the NRPB.

NOTE: These points are **not** intended to cover all aspects of the guidance notes and legislation. The various publications mentioned above, particularly the 2001 *Guidance Notes*, should be regarded as essential reading for all dental nurses, whether in general practice, dental hospitals or community clinics.

Summary of the legislation and extracts from the 2001 *Guidance Notes for Dental Practitioners on the Safe Use of X-ray Equipment*

Ionising Radiations Regulations 1999 (IRR99)

General points

- These regulations are concerned principally with the safety of workers and the general public but also address the equipment aspects of patient protection.
- They came into force on 1st January 2000.
- They replace the Ionising Radiations Regulations 1985.

Essential legal requirements

- *Authorization.* Use of dental X-ray equipment for research purposes should be in accordance with a generic authorization granted by the Health and Safety Executive (HSE).
- *Notification.* The HSE must be notified of the routine use of dental X-ray equipment and of any material changes to a notification including a change in ownership of the practice or a move to new premises.
- *Prior risk assessment.* This must be undertaken before work commences and be subject to regular review. All employers are recommended to record the findings of their risk assessment, but it is a requirement

for employers with five or more employees. A five-step approach is recommended by the HSE:

1. Identify the hazards (i.e. routine and accidental exposure to X-rays)
2. Decide who might be harmed and how they might be affected
3. Evaluate the risks and decide whether existing precautions are adequate or whether more precautions need to be taken. Implement additional precautions, if needed
4. Record the findings of the risk assessment
5. Review the risk assessment and revise it, if necessary.

- *Restriction of exposure.* There is an over-riding requirement to restrict radiation doses to staff and other persons to as low as reasonably practicable (ALARP) (see later).
- *Maintenance and examination of engineering controls.* Applies particularly to safety and warning features of dental X-ray equipment.
- *Contingency plans.* These should arise out of the risk assessment and be provided within the *Local Rules* (see later).
- *Radiation Protection Adviser (RPA).* A suitably trained RPA must be appointed in writing and consulted to give advice on IRR99. The RPA should be an expert in radiation protection and will be able to advise on compliance with the Regulations and all aspects of radiation protection, including advice on:
  — controlled and designated areas for all radiation equipment
  — installation of new or modified X-ray equipment
  — periodic examination and testing of engineering controls, safety features and warning signals
  — systems of work
  — risk assessment
  — contingency plans
  — staff training
  — assessment and recording of doses received by patients
  — quality assurance (QA) programmes.
- *Information, instruction and training.* Must be provided, as appropriate, for all persons associated with dental radiology.
- *Designated areas.* During an exposure, a *controlled area* will normally be designated

around the X-ray set as an aid to the effective control of exposures. The controlled area may be defined as within the primary X-ray beam until it has been sufficiently attenuated by distance or shielding and within 1.5 m of the X-ray tube and the patient, as shown in Figure 6.1. Normally, only the patient is allowed in this area. This can be facilitated by the use of appropriate signs, as shown in Figure 6.2.

- *Radiation Protection Supervisor (RPS)*. An RPS—usually a dentist or senior member of

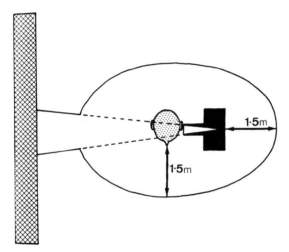

Fig. 6.1 Diagram showing the size of the *controlled area*, 1.5 m in any direction from the patient and tubehead and anywhere in the line of the main beam until it is attenuated by a solid wall.

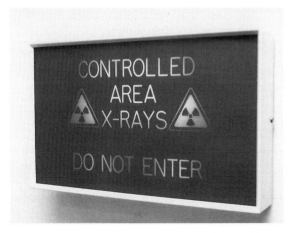

Fig. 6.2 An example of a *controlled area* warning sign. The words DO NOT ENTER are illuminated when the exposure button is pressed.

staff in the practice—should be appointed to ensure compliance with IRR99 and the *Local Rules*. The RPS must be *adequately trained*, should be closely involved with the radiography and have the authority to adequately implement their responsibilities.

- *Local Rules*. All practices should have a written set of Local Rules relating to radiation protection measures within that practice and applying to all employees. Information should include:
  — the name of the RPS
  — identification and description of the *controlled area*
  — summary of working instructions including the names of staff qualified to use the X-ray equipment and details of their training as well as instructions on the use of equipment
  — contingency arrangements in the event of equipment malfunction and/or accidental exposure to radiation
  — name of the person with legal responsibility of compliance with the regulations
  — details and results of dose-investigation levels (**Note**: A dose constraint of no higher than 1 mSv per year is recommended as generally appropriate for practice staff from dental radiography—see later section on dose limits.)
  — name and contact details of the RPA
  — arrangements for personal dosimetry
  — arrangements for pregnant staff
  — reminder to employees of their legal responsibilities under IRR99.
- *Classified persons*. Division of staff into *classified* and *non-classified* workers and the dose limits that apply to each group are discussed later. In dental practice, most staff are non-classified unless their radiography workload is very high.
- *Duties of manufacturers*. The installer is responsible for the *critical examination and report* of all new or significantly modified X-ray equipment, which should include:
  — a clear and unambiguous description of the equipment and its location
  — an evaluation of the acceptability of the location in relation to the operator's position and the room's warning signs and signals, if applicable

— an evaluation of the acceptability of the equipment's warning signals
— an evaluation of the acceptability of the exposure control
— confirmation that the equipment's safety features are in place and operating correctly (e.g. beam dimensions and alignment, beam filtration and timer operation)
— an overall conclusion as to whether or not the equipment's safety features are operating correctly, the installation is providing sufficient protection for persons from exposure to X-rays and whether the user has been provided with 'adequate information about proper use, testing and maintenance of equipment'.

• *X-ray equipment.* All equipment must be critically examined and acceptance tested before being put into clinical use and then routinely tested as part of a QA programme (see Ch. 15). The *acceptance test*, in addition to the features covered in the *critical examination* outlined above, should include:

— measurements to determine whether the equipment is operating within agreed performance parameters (e.g. operating potential (kV), X-ray output (mA) and timer accuracy (s))
— an assessment of the typical patient dose for comparison with national Diagnostic Reference Levels
— a review and record of film, film/screen combinations and processing details and an evaluation of the adequacy of processing.

A permanent record should be made of the results and conclusions of all tests and this should be retained as part of the QA programme and all deficiencies should be rectified.

All equipment (X-ray generating and image receptors) should comply with the general requirements in the regulations namely:

*Intraoral radiography
— Tube voltage should not be lower than 50 kV. New equipment should operate within the range 60–70 kV.
— All equipment should operate within 10% of the stated or selected kV setting.

— Beam diameter should not exceed 60 mm at the patient end of the spacer cone or beam-indicating device.
— Rectangular collimation (see Ch. 5) should be provided on new equipment and fitted to existing equipment at the earliest opportunity and the beam size should not exceed 40 by 50 mm.
— Total beam filtration (inherent and added) should be 1.5 mm of aluminium for sets operating below 70 kV and 2.5 mm of aluminium for sets operating above 70 kV and should be marked on the tube housing.
— The focal spot position should be marked on the outer casing of the tubehead.
— Focal spot to skin distance (FSD) should be at least 100 mm for sets operating below 60 kV and 200 mm for sets operating above 60 kV.
— Film speed controls and finely adjustable exposure time settings should be provided.
— The fastest film available (E or F speed) that will produce satisfactory diagnostic images should be used.

Panoramic radiography (see Ch. 13)
— Equipment should have a range of tube potential settings, preferably from 60 to 90 kV.
— The beam height at the receiving slit of the cassette holder should not be greater than the film in use (normally 125 mm or 150 mm). The width of the beam should not be greater than 5 mm.
— Equipment should be provided with adequate patient-positioning aids incorporating light beam markers.
— New equipment should provide facilities for field-limitation techniques.

Cephalometric radiography (see Ch. 12)
— Equipment must be able to ensure the precise alignment of X-ray beam, cassette and patient.
— The beam should be collimated to include only the diagnostically relevant area (see Ch. 12).
— To facilitate the imaging of the soft tissues, an aluminium wedge filter should be

provided at the X-ray tubehead, in preference to one at the cassette.

All equipment:

— Should have a light on the control panel to show that the mains supply is switched on.
— Should be fitted with a light that gives a clear and visible indication to the operator that an exposure is taking place and audible warnings should also provide the operator with the same information.
— Exposure switches (timers) should only function while continuous pressure is maintained on the switch and terminate if pressure is released.
— Exposure switches should be positioned so that the operator can remain outside the controlled area and at least 2 m from the X-ray tube and patient.
— Exposure times should be terminated automatically.

- *Duties of employees*. Notwithstanding the many and varied responsibilities placed on the person legally responsible, the so-called *legal person*, IRR99 places over-riding responsibilities on employees such as dental nurses which include:
  — to not knowingly expose themselves or any other person to X-rays to an extent greater than is reasonably necessary for the purposes of their work
  — to exercise reasonable care when working on any aspect of dental radiology
  — to immediately report to the *legal person* whenever they have reasonable cause to believe that an incident or accident has occurred with the X-ray equipment and that they or some other person have received an overexposure.

Ionising Radiation (Medical Exposure) Regulations 2000 (IR(ME)R 2000)

General points

- These regulations are concerned with the safety of patients.
- They came into force on 13th May 2000.
- They replace the Ionising Radiation (Protection of Persons Undergoing Medical Examination or Treatment) Regulations 1988.

- New positions of responsibility are defined, namely:
  — the employer
  — the referrer
  — the practitioner
  — the operator.

Essential legal requirements

- *Duties of employers.* The employer (*legal person*) is the person or body corporate with natural or legal responsibility for a radiological installation. He/she is responsible for providing the overall safety of the practice and for ensuring that staff and procedures conform with the regulations. In addition, the legal person must provide a framework of *written procedures* for medical exposures which should include information on:
  — procedures for correctly identifying patients before radiography
  — identification of referrers, practitioners and operators
  — authorization and justification of all clinical exposures to ensure that the justification process has taken place
  — justification of medicolegal exposures
  — identification of pregnant patients
  — compliance with and details of QA programmes
  — assessment of patient dose
  — use of diagnostic reference levels (DRLs) — defined as 'dose levels in medical radiodiagnostic practices for typical examinations for groups of standard-sized patients or standard phantoms for broadly defined types of equipment'. As such, they should not normally be exceeded without good reason. In 1999, the NRPB recommended DRLs of 4 mGy for an adult mandibular molar periapical radiograph and 65 mGy mm for an adult panoramic radiograph
  — carrying out and recording a clinical evaluation of the outcome of each exposure
  — ensuring that the probability and magnitude of accidental or unintended doses to patients are reduced as far as reasonably practicable
  — provision for carrying out clinical audits

— guidelines for referral criteria for radiographic examinations
— written protocols (guideline exposure settings) for every type of standard projection for each item of equipment
— procedures to follow if a patient is suspected of having received an excessive exposure as a result of any occurrence other than an equipment malfunction.

It is recommended that these *employers written procedures* and the *Local Rules* (see earlier) are kept together as a *radiation protection file* and that all staff are made aware of the contents.

- *Duties of the Practitioner, Operator and Referrer.*
The referrer: a registered doctor or dentist or other health professional entitled to refer a patient to a *practitioner* for a medical exposure. The *referrer* is responsible for supplying the *practitioner* with sufficient information to justify an appropriate exposure.
The practitioner: a registered doctor or dentist or other health professional entitled to take responsibility for a medical exposure. The *practitioner* must be adequately trained to take decisions and the responsibility for the justification of every exposure.
The operator: the person conducting any practical aspect of a medical exposure. Practical aspects include:
  * patient identification
  * positioning the film, patient or X-ray tubehead
  * setting the exposure parameters
  * pressing the exposure switch to initiate the exposure
  * processing films
  * clinical evaluation of radiographs
  * exposing test objects as part of the QA programme.
  The *operator* must be adequately trained for his/her role in the exposure (see later).
- *Justification of individual medical exposures.*
Before an exposure can take place, it must be justified (i.e. assessed to ensure that it will lead to a change in the patient's management and prognosis) by an *IRMER practitioner* and authorized as the means of demonstrating that it has been justified. Every exposure should be justified on the grounds of:

— the availability and/or findings of previous radiographs
— the specific objectives of the exposure in relation to the history and examination of the patient
— the total potential diagnostic benefit to the patient
— the radiation risk associated with the radiographic examination
— the efficacy, benefits and risks of alternative techniques having the same objective but involving no or less exposure to ionizing radiation.

Note: The 1998 *Selection Criteria in Dental Radiography* (see later) states that there can be no possible justification for the routine radiography of 'new' patients prior to clinical examination. A history and clinical examination are the only acceptable means of determining that the most appropriate, or necessary, radiographic views are requested.

- *Optimization.* All doses must be kept as low as reasonably practicable (ALARP) consistent with the intended purpose. This includes the need to apply QA procedures to the optimization of patient dose (see Ch. 15).
- *Clinical audit.* Provisions must be made for clinical audit. Suitable topics could include the various aspects of the QA programme (see Ch. 15), the appropriateness of radiographic requests and the clinical evaluation of radiographs.
- *Expert advice.* The regulations lay down the need for, and involvement of a Medical Physics Expert (MPE) who would give advice on such matters as the measurement and optimization of patient dose. However, the need for medical physics support in dental practice is fairly limited and in most cases the RPA should be able to act as the MPE.
- *Equipment.* The keeping and maintenance of an up-to-date inventory of each item of equipment is required and should include:
— name of manufacturer
— model number
— serial number or other unique identifier
— year of manufacture
— year of installation.

- *Adequate training and continuing education.* *Operators* and *practitioners* must have received adequate training and must undertake continuing education and training after qualification. The nature of this training is then specified in the *Guidance Notes*:

  — **Adequate training for UK graduated practitioners:**
  An undergraduate degree conforming to the requirements for the undergraduate curriculum in dental radiology and imaging as specified by the General Dental Council and including the core curriculum in dental radiography and radiology as specified in the NRPB/RCR 1994 *Guidelines on Radiology Standards in Primary Dental Care.*

  — **Adequate training for operators involved in selecting exposure settings and/or positioning the patient, film or X-ray tubehead:**
    ⋆ *Dentists — practitioner* training (as above)
    ⋆ *Dental nurses —* should possess the Certificate in Dental Radiography from a course conforming to the syllabus prescribed by the College of Radiographers (although interim measures allow some flexibility in these requirements until 2005)
    ⋆ *Dental hygienists and therapists —* should have received an equivalent level of training to that for dental nurses.

  — **Adequate training for other operators**:
  Dental nurses and other such operators should preferably possess the Certificate in Dental Nursing or they must have received adequate and documented training specific to the tasks that they undertake. Dental nurses (or other staff), who simply 'press the exposure button' after the patient has been prepared by another adequately trained *operator*, may only do so in the continued presence and under the direct supervision of that *operator.*

  — **Continuing education and training for practitioners:**
  Continuing education and training in all aspects of dental radiology should be part of *practitioners* and *operators* life-long learning. To this end, it is recommended

  that *practitioners* attend a formal course (equivalent to 5 hours of verifiable continuing education) every 5 years covering all aspects of radiation protection including:
    ⋆ principles of radiation physics
    ⋆ risks of ionizing radiation
    ⋆ radiation doses in dental radiography
    ⋆ factors affecting doses in dental radiography
    ⋆ principles of radiation protection
    ⋆ statutory requirements
    ⋆ selection criteria
    ⋆ quality assurance.

  — **Continuing education for operators involved in radiographing patients:**
  These *operators* are also recommended to attend a continuing education course every 5 years that covers:
    ⋆ principles of radiation physics
    ⋆ risks of ionizing radiation
    ⋆ radiation doses in dental radiography
    ⋆ factors affecting doses in dental radiography
    ⋆ principles of radiation protection
    ⋆ statutory requirements
    ⋆ quality assurance.

- *Lead protection.* The confusion and controversy which surrounded the use of lead protection was the main instigating factor in the 1994 NRPB/RCR guidelines. They concluded that patient protection was best achieved by implementation of practical dose reduction measures in relation to clinical judgement, equipment and radiographic technique and not by lead protection. This view has been endorsed in the 2001 *Guidance Notes* which state:

  — There is no justification for the routine use of lead aprons for patients in dental radiography.
  — Thyroid collars, as shown in Figure 6.3, should be used in those few cases where the thyroid may be in primary beam. (In the author's opinion, this can include maxillary occlusal radiography, and thyroid protection is therefore shown in Chapter 10.)
  — Lead aprons do not protect against radiation scattered internally within the

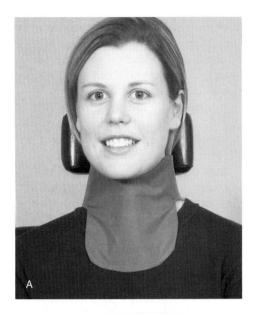

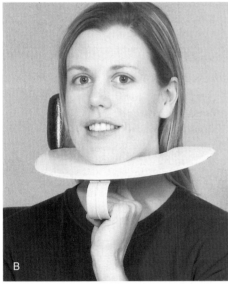

Fig. 6.3 Examples of thyroid lead protection. **A** Lead collar (0.5 mm Pb equivalent). **B** Hand-held neck shield (0.5 mm Pb equivalent).

body, and only provide a practicable degree of protection in the case of the infrequently used vertex occlusal projection. Even in this case, the use of the lead apron could only be regarded as prudent for a female patient who is, or may be, pregnant.

— Protective aprons, having a lead equivalence of not less than 0.25 mm, should be provided for any adult who provides assistance by supporting a patient during radiography.

— When a lead apron is provided, it must be correctly stored (e.g. over a suitable hanger) and not folded. Its condition must be routinely checked including a visual inspection at annual intervals.

Specific requirements for women of childbearing age.
The developing fetus is most susceptible to the dangers of ionizing radiation during the period of organogenesis (2–9 weeks) — often before the woman knows that she is pregnant. IR(ME)R2000 prohibits the carrying out of a medical exposure of a female of childbearing age without an enquiry as to whether she is pregnant **if** the primary beam is likely to irradiate the pelvic area. This is highly unlikely in dental radiography. Even so, it is recommended, essentially for psychological reasons, that the operator should enquire of all women of childbearing age whether they are pregnant or likely to be pregnant. If the answer is yes, then, in addition to the routine protective measures appropriate for all patients, the following specific points should be considered:

— The justification should be reviewed to ensure that only radiographs that are absolutely necessary are taken, e.g. delay routine periodic checks.
— The patient should be reassured that a minimal dose is being employed and the patient given the option to delay the radiography.
— As mentioned earlier, it may be prudent to use a protective lead apron when taking the infrequently used *vertex occlusal* projection.

Dose limitation and annual dose limits

For the purposes of dose limitation, the ICRP has divided the population into three groups:

- Patients
- Radiation workers (classified and non-classified)
- General public.

Patients

Radiographic investigations involving patients are divided into four subgroups:

- Examinations directly associated with illness
- Systematic examinations (periodic health checks)
- Examinations for occupational, medicolegal or insurance purposes
- Examinations for medical research.

Examinations directly associated with illness

- There are no set dose limits.
- The decision to carry out such an investigation should be based on:
  — A correct assessment of the indications
  — The expected yield
  — The way in which the results are likely to influence the diagnosis and subsequent treatment
  — The clinician having an adequate knowledge of the physical properties and biological effects of ionizing radiation (i.e. *adequately trained*).
- The number, type and frequency of the radiographs requested or taken (selection criteria) are the responsibility of the clinician. Selection criteria recommendations have been published in different countries in recent years to provide guidance in this clinical area of radiation protection. In the UK, the *Selection Criteria in Dental Radiography* booklet was published in 1998 by the Faculty of General Dental Practitioners of the Royal College of Surgeons of England and, as stated earlier, should be regarded as recommended reading for all dental nurses. The expert group responsible for this document reviewed the available scientific evidence to formulate evidence-based recommendations as far as was possible. In some areas, where scientific evidence was lacking, their recommendations were based on expert clinical opinion. The overview of their recommendations is reproduced in Table 6.1.

Systematic examinations (periodic health checks)

- There are no set dose limits.
- There should be a high probability of obtaining useful information—see *Selection Criteria* recommendations in Table 6.1.
- The information obtained should be important to the patient's health.

Examinations for occupational, medicolegal or insurance purposes

- There are no set dose limits.
- The benefit is primarily to a third party.
- The patient should at least benefit indirectly.
- The 2001 *Guidance Notes* emphasize that the need for, and the usefulness of, these examinations should be critically examined when assessing whether they are justified. They also recommend that these types of examinations should only be requested by medical/dental practitioners and that the patient's consent should be obtained.

Examinations for medical research

- There are no set dose limits.
- All research projects should be approved on the advice of an appropriate expert group or Ethics Committee and subject to Local Rules and regulations.
- All volunteers should have a full understanding of the risks involved and give their consent.

Radiation workers

Radiation workers are those people who are exposed to radiation during the course of their work. This exposure carries no benefit only risk. The ICRP further divides these workers into two subgroups depending on the level of occupational exposure:

- Classified workers
- Non-classified workers.

Table 6.1 Overview of the recommendations from the 1998 *Selection Criteria in Dental Radiography*. N.B. No radiographs should be taken without a history and clinical examination having been performed (Reproduced with kind permission from the Faculty of General Dental Practitioners of the Royal College of Surgeons of England.)

Patient category		Dentate individuals				Endentulous
	SELECTION CRITERIA	CHILD – PRIMARY DENTITION	CHILD – MIXED DENTITION	ADOLESCENT	ADULTS	
NEW PATIENT	All new patients to assess dental diseases and growth and development	Posterior bitewing examination as indicated after clinical examination	Patient-specific radiographic examination as indicated after clinical assessment	Patient-specific radiographic examination consisting of posterior bitewings and selected periapicals. An extensive intraoral radiographic examination may be appropriate when the patient presents with clinical evidence of generalized dental disease or a history of extensive dental treatment. Alternatively, a panoramic radiograph may be appropriate in some instances		Periapical radiograph/s of any symptomatic or clinically suspicious areas
	Growth and development	Not normally indicated	Patient-specific radiographic examination as indicated after clinical assessment	One-off periapical or panoramic examination to assess development of third molars if **symptomatic**		Not normally indicated
RECALL PATIENT	High Caries Risk	**Posterior bitewing examinations at 6-month intervals* or until no new or progressing carious lesions are evident** *Bitewings should not be taken more frequently and it is imperative to reassess caries risk in order to justify using this interval again.				Not applicable
	Moderate Caries Risk†	Posterior bitewing examinations at 1-year intervals				Not applicable
	Low Caries Risk	Posterior bitewing examination at 12 – 18 month intervals	**Posterior bitewing examination at 2-year intervals. more extended radiographic recall intervals may be employed if there is explicit evidence of continuing low caries risk.**			Not applicable
	Periodontal disease or history of periodontal disease	Patient-specific radiographic examination of selected periapical and/or bitewings for areas where periodontal disease (other than non-specific gingivitis) can be demonstrated clinically				Not applicable

†Re-assess caries risk at each visit

Table 6.2 The previous annual dose limits and those currently in force under the Ionising Radiations Regulations 1999

	Old dose limits	New dose limits (IRR99)
Classified workers	50 mSv	20 mSv
Non-classified workers	15 mSv	6 mSv
General public	5 mSv	1 mSv

The ICRP sets maximum dose limits for each group, based on the principle that the risk to any worker who receives the full dose limit, will be such that the worker will be at no greater risk than a worker in another hazardous, but non-radioactive, environment. The annual dose limits have been revised under the Ionising Radiations Regulations 1999 and these are shown in Table 6.2.

The main features of each group of radiation workers are summarized below:

Classified workers

- Receive high levels of exposure to radiation at work (if *Local Rules* are observed this is highly unlikely in dental practice).
- Require compulsory personal monitoring.
- Require compulsory annual health checks.

Non-classified workers (most dental staff)

- Receive low levels of exposure to radiation at work (as in the dental surgery).
- The annual dose limits are 3/10 of the classified workers' limits. Provided the *Local Rules* are observed, all dental staff should receive an annual effective dose of considerably less than the limit of 6 mSv. Hence, the regulations suggest the setting of 'Dose Constraints'. These represent the upper level of individual dose that should not be exceeded in a well-managed practice and for dental radiography the following recommendations are made:

1 mSv	for employees directly involved with the radiography (operators)
0.3 mSv	for employees not directly involved with the radiography and for members of the general public.

In addition to the above dose limits, the legal person must ensure that the dose to the fetus of any pregnant member of staff is unlikely to exceed 1 mSv during the declared term of the pregnancy.

- Personal monitoring (see later) is not compulsory, although it is recommended if the risk assessment indicates that individual doses could exceed 1 mSv per year. The 2001 *Guidance Notes* state that in practice this should be considered for those staff whose weekly workload exceeds 100 intraoral or 50 panoramic films, or a pro-rata combination of each type of examination.
- Annual health checks are not required.

The radiation dose to dentists and their staff can come from:

- The primary beam, if they stand in its path
- Scattered radiation from the patient
- Radiation leakage from the tubehead.

The main protective measures to limit the dose that workers might receive are therefore based mainly on a combination of common sense and the knowledge that ionizing radiation is attenuated by distance and obeys the inverse square law (see Fig. 6.4).

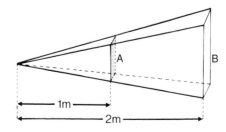

Fig. 6.4 Diagrammatic representation of the inverse square law. Doubling the distance from the source means that the area of B is four times the area of A, thus the radiation per unit area at B is one quarter that at A. (Reproduced with kind permission of Mr B. Beeching.)

The main dose limitation measures relate to:

- Distance from the source of radiation—staff should stand outside the *controlled area* (see Fig. 6.1) and not in the line of the primary beam. If these positions cannot be obtained, appropriate lead screens/barriers should be used
- Safe use of equipment—as summarized in the 2001 *Guidance Notes*
- Radiographic technique—staff should be adequately trained and follow the recommendations summarized in the 2001 *Guidance Notes*
- Monitoring (see later).

General public

This group includes everyone who is not receiving a radiation dose either as a patient or as a radiation worker, but who may be exposed inadvertently, for example, someone in a dental surgery waiting room, in other rooms in the building or passers-by. The annual dose limits for this group have been lowered to 1 mSv, as shown in Table 6.2 although the suggested 'Dose Constraint' is 0.3 mSv (see earlier). The general public are at risk from the primary beam, so specific consideration should be given to:

- The siting of X-ray equipment to ensure that the primary beam is not aimed directly into occupied rooms or corridors
- The thickness/material of partitioning walls
- Advice from the RPA (see 1999 Regulations) on the siting of all X-ray equipment, surgery design and the placement of radiation warning signs.

Main methods of monitoring and measuring radiation dose

There are three main devices (shown in Fig. 6.5), for monitoring and measuring radiation dose:

- Film badges
- Thermoluminescent dosemeters (TLD)
  — Badge
  — Extremity monitor

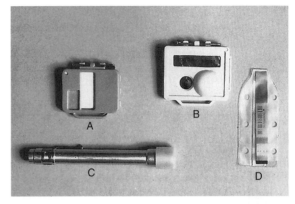

Fig. 6.5 Monitoring devices. **A** Personal monitoring film badge. **B** Personal monitoring TLD badge. **C** Ionization bleeper. **D** TLD extremity monitor.

- Ionization chambers.

Film badges

The main features of film badges are:

- They consist of a blue plastic frame containing a variety of different metal filters and a small radiographic film which reacts to radiation
- They are worn on the outside of the clothes, usually at the level of the reproductive organs, for 1–3 months before being processed
- They are the most common form of personal monitoring device currently in use.

Advantages

- Provides a permanent record of dose received.
- May be checked and reassessed at a later date.
- Can measure the type and energy of radiation encountered.
- Simple, robust and relatively inexpensive.

Disadvantages

- No immediate indication of exposure — all information is retrospective.
- Processing is required which may lead to errors.
- The badges are prone to filter loss.

Thermoluminescent dosemeters

The main features of TLDs are:

- They are used for personal monitoring of the whole body and/or the extremities, as well as measuring the skin dose from particular investigations
- They contain materials such as lithium fluoride (LiF) which absorb radiation and then release the energy in the form of light when heated
- The intensity of the emitted light is proportional to the radiation energy absorbed originally
- Personal monitors consist of a yellow or orange plastic holder, worn like the film badge for 1–3 months.

Advantages

- The lithium fluoride is re-usable.
- Read-out measurements are easily automated and rapidly produced.
- Suitable for a wide variety of dose measurements.

Disadvantages

- Read-out is destructive, giving no permanent record, results cannot be checked or reassessed.

- Only limited information provided on the type and energy of the radiation.
- Dose gradients are not detectable.
- Relatively expensive.

Ionization chambers

The main features of ionization chambers are:

- They are used for personal monitoring (thimble chamber) and by physicists (free-air chamber) to measure radiation exposure
- Radiation produces ionization of the air molecules inside the closed chamber, which results in a measurable discharge and hence a direct read-out
- They are available in many different sizes and forms.

Advantages

- The most accurate method of measuring radiation dose.
- Direct read-out gives immediate information.

Disadvantages

- They give no permanent record of exposure.
- No indication of the type or energy of the radiation.
- Personal ionization monitors are not very sensitive to low-energy radiation.
- They are fragile and easily damaged.

Radiography

Dental radiography— general patient considerations including control of infection

This short chapter is designed as a preface to the radiography section. It summarizes the general guidelines relating to patient care, pertinent to all aspects of dental radiography, thus avoiding unnecessary repetition in subsequent chapters. Measures aimed at the control of infection during radiography are also discussed.

General guidelines on patient care

- For intraoral radiography the patient should be positioned comfortably in the dental chair, ideally with the occlusal plane horizontal and parallel to the floor. For most projections the head should be supported against the chair to minimize unwanted movement. This upright positioning is assumed in subsequent chapters when describing radiographic techniques. However, some operators elect to X-ray their patients in the supine position along with most other dental surgery procedures. All techniques need to be modified accordingly, but it can sometimes be more difficult to assess angulations and achieve accurate alignment of film and tubehead with the patient lying down.
- For extraoral views the patient should be reassured about the large, possibly frightening or unfriendly-looking equipment, before being positioned within the machine. This is of particular importance with children.
- The procedure should be explained to the patients in terms they can understand, including warning them not to move during the investigation.
- Spectacles, dentures or orthodontic appliances should be removed. Jewellery including ear-

rings may also need to be removed for certain projections.
- A protective lead thyroid collar, if deemed appropriate for the investigation being carried out, should be placed on the patient (see Ch. 6).
- The exposure factors on the control panel should be selected before positioning the intraoral film packet and X-ray tubehead, in order to reduce the time of any discomfort associated with the investigation.
- Intraoral film packets should be positioned carefully to avoid trauma to the soft tissues taking particular care where tissues curve, e.g. the anterior hard palate, lingual to the mandibular incisor teeth and distolingual to the mandibular molars.
- The radiographic investigation should be carried out as accurately and as quickly as possible, to avoid having to retake the radiograph and to lessen patient discomfort.
- The patient should always be watched throughout the exposure to check that he/she has obeyed instructions and has not moved.

Specific requirements when X-raying children and patients with disabilities

These two groups of patients can present particular problems during radiography, including:

- Difficulty in obtaining cooperation
- Anatomical difficulties, such as:
  — large tongue (macroglossia)
  — small mouth (microstomia)

— tight oral musculature
— limited neck movement
— narrow dental arches
— shallow palate
— obesity.

- Neurological disabilities, such as:
— communication and learning difficulties
— tremor
— palsy.

As a result of these difficulties, the following additional guidelines should be considered:

- Only radiographic investigations appropriate to the limitations imposed by the patient's age, cooperation or disability should be attempted
- Select intraoral films of appropriate size, modifying standard techniques as necessary
- Utilize assistant(s) to help hold the film and/or steady and reassure the patient. This can be accomplished by using an accompanying relative, rather than repeatedly using a member of staff.

NOTE: In the UK, the Ionizing Radiations Regulations 1999 require that during an exposure a designated *controlled area* must exist around the X-ray set and theoretically only the patient is allowed in this area (see Ch. 6). Therefore, if assistance is needed and this requirement cannot be fulfilled, the *radiation protection adviser* (RPA) must advise on the appropriate protective measures for the assistant.

- Perform any necessary radiography under general anaesthesia, if an uncooperative patient is having their dental treatment in this manner (see Fig. 7.1). Radiographs taken are usually restricted to oblique laterals and periapicals although bitewings can be taken.

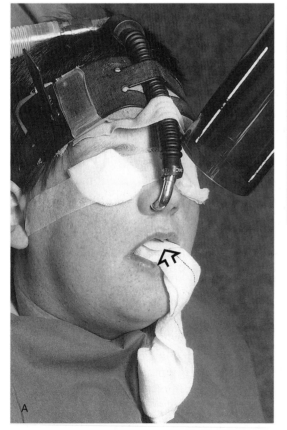
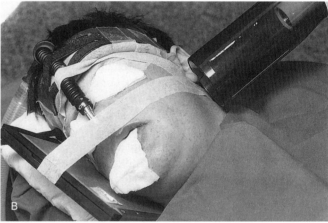

Fig. 7.1 Patient positioning for radiography under general anaesthesia. **A** Periapical radiography of upper incisor teeth. Note the film packet (arrowed) supported in the desired position by a gauze pack. **B** Oblique lateral radiography. Note the tape used to stabilize the cassette and maintain the correct patient position. (Kindly provided by Mr P. Erridge.)

- Avoid dental panoramic tomography because of the need for the patient to remain still for approximately 18 seconds (see Ch. 13). Oblique lateral radiographs should be regarded as the extraoral views of choice.
- Use the paralleling technique, if possible, for periapical radiography because with this technique the relative positions of the film packet, teeth and X-ray beam are maintained, irrespective of the position of the patient's head (see Ch. 8).

Control of infection

In the UK, The Health and Safety at Work, Etc, Act of 1974 states that every person working in hospitals or general practice (referred to as *health care workers* or HCWs) has a legal duty to ensure that all necessary steps are taken to prevent cross-infection to protect themselves, their colleagues and the patients. In addition, The Management of Health and Safety Regulations 1992 requires that a risk assessment is carried out for all procedures to reduce the possibility of harm to staff and patients. Effective infection control measures are therefore required in dental radiography even though most investigations are regarded as *non-invasive* or *non-exposure prone procedures*, because they do not involve breaches of the mucosa or skin. The main risk of cross-infection is from one patient to another from salivary contamination of work areas and equipment. HCWs themselves are not at great risk during radiography but there are no grounds for complacency.

Main infections of concern

- *Infective hepatitis caused by hepatitis B (HBV) or hepatitis C (HCV) viruses.* The WHO estimates that of the 2 billion people that have been infected with HBV, more than 350 million have chronic (lifelong) infections. In the developing world, 8% to 10% of people in the general population become chronically infected. HBV is thought to be 50 to 100 times more infectious than HIV. The WHO estimates that 3% of the world's population has been infected with HCV.

- *Human immunodeficiency virus (HIV disease and AIDS caused by HIV)*.
- *Tuberculosis (TB)*. The incidence of all forms of TB is rising and now approximately one-third of the world's population is infected. Many of the people with active TB are also infected with HIV.
- *Cold sores caused by herpes simplex virus (HSV)*. HCWs are at risk of getting herpetic whitlow, a painful finger infection.
- *Rubella (German measles)*.
- *Syphilis*.
- *Diphtheria*.
- *Mumps*.
- *Influenza*.
- *Transmissible spongiform encephalopathies* (TSEs), e.g. Creutzfeldt–Jakob disease (CJD).

A thorough medical history should therefore be obtained from all patients. However, the medical history and examination may not identify asymptomatic carriers of infectious diseases.

It is therefore safer for HCWs to accept that ALL patients may be an infection risk — age or class is no barrier — and universal precautions should be adopted. This means that the same infection control measures should be used for all patients, the only exception being for patients known to have or suspected of having TSEs and the small number of patients in the defined risk groups for TSEs.

Important point to note

If dental clinicians are requesting other HCWs to take their radiographs, either in hospitals or general dental practice, it is their responsibility to ensure that these workers are made aware of any known medical problems or risks, e.g. epilepsy or current infections.

Infection control measures

As mentioned previously, in dental radiography the main concerns arise from salivary contamination of work areas and equipment. Suitable precautions include:

- Training of all staff in infection control procedures and monitoring their compliance.

- All clinical staff should be vaccinated against hepatitis B, have their response to this vaccine checked and maintain this vaccination.
- Open wounds on the hands should be covered with waterproof dressings.
- Latex or vinyl non-sterile, non-powdered medical gloves should be worn for all radiographic procedures and changed after every patient.
- Eye protection — either safety glasses or visors (see Fig. 7.2) should be worn but masks are not usually necessary for radiography.
- All required film packets and holders should be placed on disposable trays to avoid contamination of work surfaces.
- To prevent salivary contamination of film packets, they can be placed in small barrier envelopes or preferably purchased pre-packed in such envelopes, before use (see Fig. 7.3). After being used in the mouth, the film packet can be emptied out of the barrier envelope onto a clean surface and then handled safely.

- Digital radiography sensors must also be placed inside appropriate barrier envelopes (see Fig. 7.4).
- If barrier envelopes are not used, saliva should be wiped from exposed film packets with disinfectant (e.g. 1% hypochlorite) before handling and processing. This is of particular importance if daylight-loading automatic processors are used because of the risk of salivary contamination of the soft flexible arm sleeves (see Ch. 5 and Fig. 5.24), and if films are collected together during the course of the working day and then processed in batches.
- Film packets must only be introduced into daylight-loading processors using clean hands or washed gloves. Powdered gloves may cause artefacts on the films.
- Contaminated disposable trays, barrier envelopes and film packaging should be discarded directly into suitable clinical waste disposal bags.

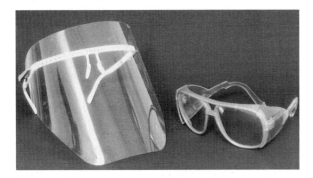

Fig. 7.2 Plastic safety glasses and Vista-Tec visor (Polydentia SA) suitable for eye protection during dental radiography.

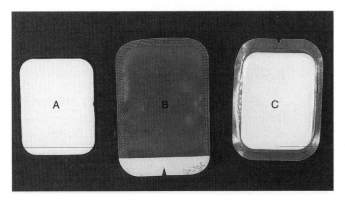

Fig. 7.3 A 31 × 41 mm periapical film packet. **B** Plastic barrier envelope to take the periapical film. **C** Pre-packed periapical film packet inside its barrier envelope.

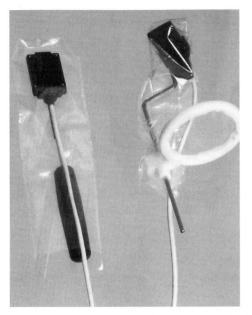

Fig. 7.4 CCD digital sensors in holders covered by plastic barrier envelopes.

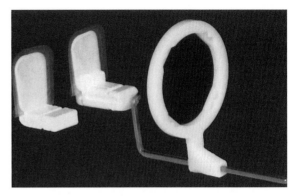

Fig. 7.5 Rinn disposable polystyrene bite blocks for both paralleling and bisected angle technique periapicals.

- All film holders/bite blocks/bite pegs should be washed after use and then autoclaved or discarded, if disposable.
- X-ray equipment, including the tubehead, control panel, timer switch and cassettes which have been touched during the radiographic procedure should be wiped after each patient with a suitable surface disinfectant, e.g. Mikrozid®.
- Alternatively, all pieces of equipment can be covered, for example with cling film, which can be replaced after every patient.
- Soiled gloves and cleaning swabs should be placed in suitable disposal bags and sealed for incineration.

Important points to note

- When X-raying known or suspected TSE patients, extraoral radiographic techniques, that avoid salivary contamination, should be chosen whenever possible (preferably using a technique that does not involve any form of intraoral positioning device) and films should be processed immediately and not left on work surfaces.
- If intraoral techniques are necessary, disposable film holders should be used (see Fig. 7.5).

Footnote

The importance of effective control of infection measures during dental radiography cannot be over-emphasized. All health care workers should remember that they have a duty of care to do no harm to their patients. Inadequate infection control measures may put other/subsequent patients at risk from infection whether transmitted directly or indirectly.

8 Periapical radiography

Periapical radiography describes intraoral techniques designed to show individual teeth and the tissues *around the apices*. Each film usually shows two to four teeth and provides detailed information about the teeth and the surrounding alveolar bone.

Main indications

The main clinical indications for periapical radiography include:

- Detection of apical infection/inflammation
- Assessment of the periodontal status
- After trauma to the teeth and associated alveolar bone
- Assessment of the presence and position of unerupted teeth
- Assessment of root morphology before extractions
- During endodontics
- Preoperative assessment and postoperative appraisal of apical surgery
- Detailed evaluation of apical cysts and other lesions within the alveolar bone
- Evaluation of implants postoperatively.

Ideal positioning requirements

The ideal requirements for the position of the film packet and the X-ray beam, relative to a tooth, are shown in Figure 8.1. They include:

- The tooth under investigation and the film packet should be in contact or, if not feasible, as close together as possible
- The tooth and the film packet should be parallel to one another

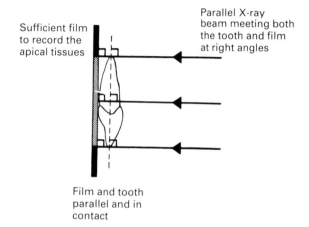

Sufficient film to record the apical tissues

Parallel X-ray beam meeting both the tooth and film at right angles

Film and tooth parallel and in contact

Fig. 8.1 Diagram illustrating the ideal geometrical relationship between film, tooth and X-ray beam.

- The film packet should be positioned with its long axis vertically for incisors and canines, and horizontally for premolars and molars with sufficient film beyond the apices to record the apical tissues
- The X-ray tubehead should be positioned so that the beam meets the tooth and the film at right angles in both the vertical and the horizontal planes
- The positioning should be reproducible.

Radiographic techniques

The anatomy of the oral cavity does not always allow all these ideal positioning requirements to be satisfied. In an attempt to overcome the problems, two techniques for periapical radiography have been developed:

- The paralleling technique
- The bisected angle technique.

Paralleling technique

Theory

1. The film packet is placed in a holder and positioned in the mouth **parallel** to the long axis of the tooth under investigation.

2. The X-ray tubehead is then aimed at right angles (vertically and horizontally) to both the tooth and the film packet.

3. By using a film holder with fixed film packet and X-ray tubehead positions, the technique is reproducible.

This positioning has the potential to satisfy four of the five ideal requirements mentioned earlier.

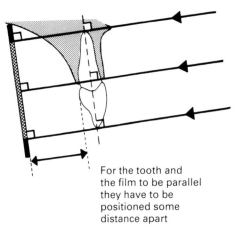

For the tooth and the film to be parallel they have to be positioned some distance apart

Fig. 8.2 Diagram showing the position the film packet has to occupy in the mouth to be parallel to the long axis of the tooth, because of the slope of the palate.

However, the anatomy of the palate and the shape of the arches mean that the tooth and the film packet cannot be both parallel and in contact. As shown in Figure 8.2, the film packet has to be positioned some distance from the tooth.

To prevent the magnification of the image that this separation would cause, a parallel, non-diverging, X-ray beam is required (see Fig. 8.3). As explained in Chapter 5, this is achieved usually by having a large *focal spot to skin distance*, by having a **long spacer cone** or beam-indicating device (BID) on the X-ray set.

Film packet holders

A variety of holders has been developed for this technique. The choice of holder is a matter of personal preference — the Rinn XCP® holders, shown in Figure 8.4, being favoured by the author. The different holders vary in cost and design but essentially consist of three basic components:

- A mechanism for holding the film packet parallel to the teeth that also prevents bending of the packet
- A bite block or platform
- An X-ray beam-aiming device. This may or may not provide additional collimation of the beam.

Positioning techniques

The radiographic techniques for the permanent dentition can be summarized as follows:

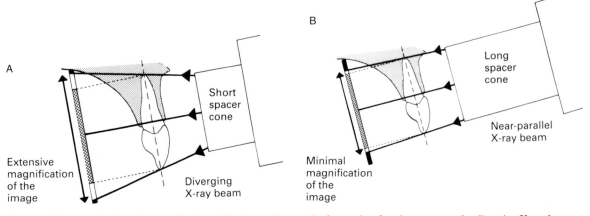

A

Short spacer cone

Extensive magnification of the image

Diverging X-ray beam

B

Long spacer cone

Near-parallel X-ray beam

Minimal magnification of the image

Fig. 8.3 Diagrams showing the magnification of the image that results from using **A** a short cone and a diverging X-ray beam and **B** a long cone and a near-parallel X-ray beam.

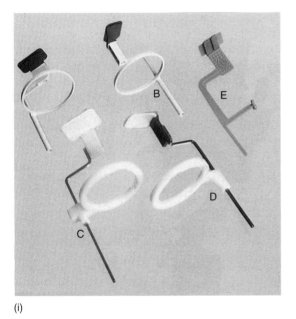

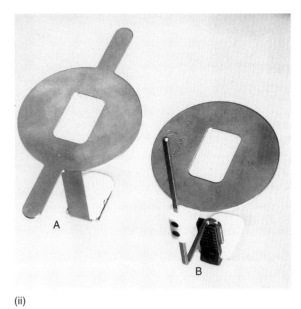

(i)   (ii)

Fig. 8.4 (i) A selection of film packet holders designed for the paralleling technique. **A** Hawe–Neos Superbite posterior holder (colour coded red). **B** Hawe–Neos Superbite anterior holder (colour coded green). **C** Rinn XCP posterior holder (colour coded yellow). **D** Rinn XCP anterior holder (colour coded blue) with film packet inserted. **E** Unibite® posterior holder. **(ii)** Rectangular collimation provided by **A** the Masel Precision all-in-one metal holder and **B** the Rinn XCP holder with its additional metal collimator attached to the white locator ring.

1. The appropriate holder and size of film packet are selected. *For incisors and canines* (maxillary and mandibular) an anterior holder should be used and a small film packet (22 × 35 mm) with its long axis vertical. For *premolars and molars* (maxillary and mandibular) use a posterior holder (right or left as required) and a large film packet (31 × 41 mm) with its long axis horizontal, in addition:

    a. The smooth, white surface of the film packet must face towards the X-ray tubehead.

    b. The end of the film packet with the embossed orientation dot is placed opposite the **crowns** of the teeth (to avoid subsequent superimposition of the dot over an apex).

2. The patient is positioned with the head supported and with the occlusal plane horizontal.

3. The holder and film packet are placed in the mouth as follows:

    a. *Maxillary incisors and canines* — the film packet is positioned sufficiently posteriorly to enable its height to be accommodated in the vault of the palate

    b. *Mandibular incisors and canines* — the film packet is positioned in the floor of the

mouth, approximately in line with the lower canines or first premolars

    c. *Maxillary premolars and molars* — the film packet is placed in the midline of the palate, again to accommodate its height in the vault of the palate

    d. *Mandibular premolars and molars* — the film packet is placed in the lingual sulcus next to the appropriate teeth.

4. The holder is rotated so that the teeth under investigation are touching the bite block.

5. A cottonwool roll is placed on the reverse side of the bite block. This often helps to keep the tooth and film packet parallel and may make the holder less uncomfortable.

6. The patient is requested to bite **gently** together, to stabilize the holder in position.

7. The locator ring is moved down the indicator rod until it is just in contact with the patient's face. This ensures the correct focal spot to film distance.

8. The spacer cone or BID is aligned with the locator ring. This automatically sets the vertical and horizontal angles and centres the X-ray beam on the film packet.

9. The exposure is made (see Figs 8.5–8.12).

Maxillary incisors

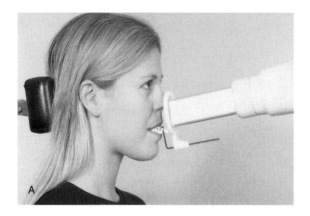

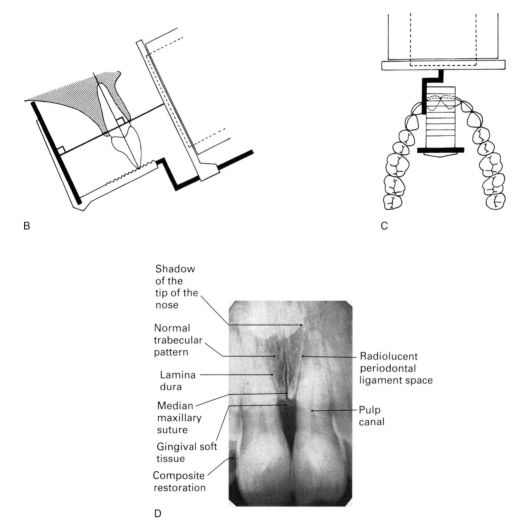

Shadow of the tip of the nose

Normal trabecular pattern

Lamina dura

Median maxillary suture

Gingival soft tissue

Composite restoration

Radiolucent periodontal ligament space

Pulp canal

Fig. 8.5A Patient positioning (Maxillary central incisor). **B** Diagram of the positioning. **C** Plan view of the positioning. **D** Resultant radiograph with the main radiographic features indicated.

Maxillary canine

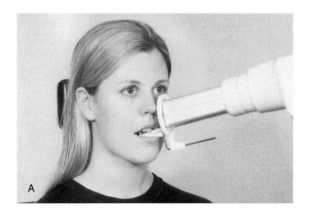

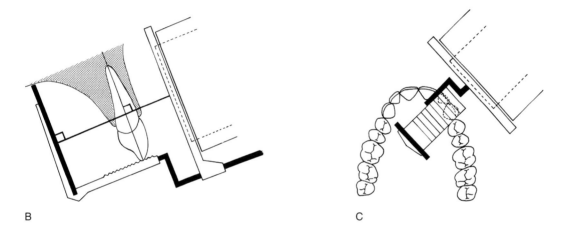

B   C

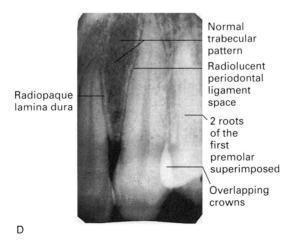

Radiopaque
lamina dura

Normal
trabecular
pattern

Radiolucent
periodontal
ligament
space

2 roots
of the
first
premolar
superimposed

Overlapping
crowns

D

Fig. 8.6A Patient positioning (Maxillary canine). **B** Diagram of the positioning. **C** Plan view of the positioning. **D** Resultant radiograph with the main radiographic features indicated.

Maxillary premolars

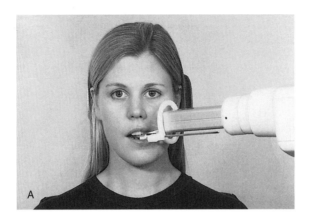

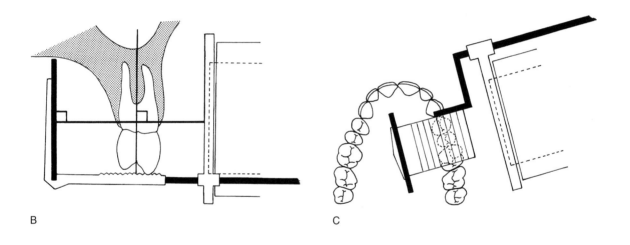

B   C

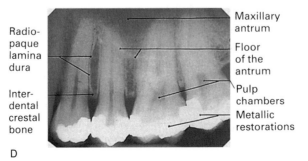

Radio-
paque
lamina
dura

Inter-
dental
crestal
bone

Maxillary
antrum

Floor
of the
antrum

Pulp
chambers

Metallic
restorations

D

Fig. 8.7A Patient positioning (Maxillary premolars). **B** Diagram of the positioning. **C** Plan view of the positioning. **D** Resultant radiograph with the main radiographic features indicated.

Maxillary molars

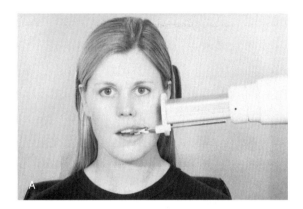

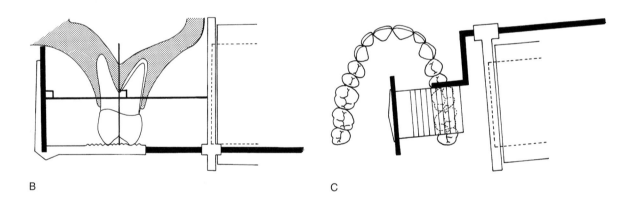

B   C

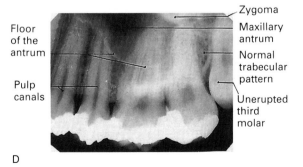

Zygoma

Floor
of the
antrum

Maxillary
antrum

Normal
trabecular
pattern

Pulp
canals

Unerupted
third
molar

D

Fig. 8.8A Patient positioning (Maxillary molars). **B** Diagram of the positioning. **C** Plan view of the positioning. **D** Resultant radiograph with the main radiographic features indicated.

Mandibular incisors

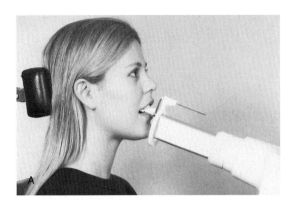

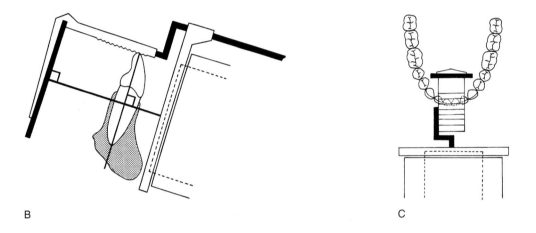

B

C

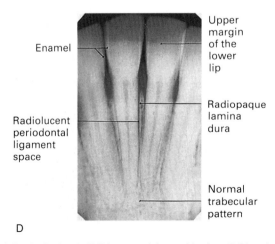

Enamel

Upper
margin
of the
lower
lip

Radiolucent
periodontal
ligament
space

Radiopaque
lamina
dura

Normal
trabecular
pattern

D

Fig. 8.9A Patient positioning (Mandibular incisors). **B** Diagram of the positioning. **C** Plan view of the positioning. **D** Resultant radiograph with the main radiographic features indicated.

Mandibular canine

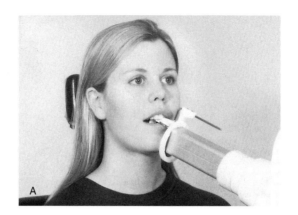

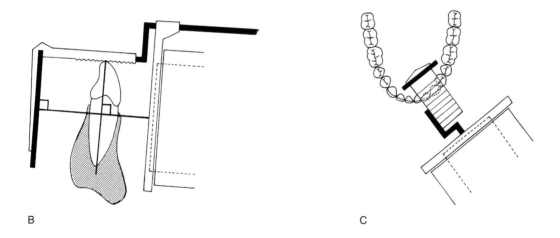

B

C

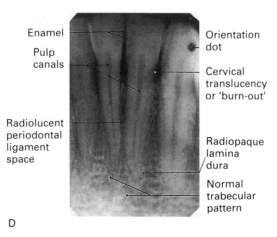

D

Fig. 8.10A Patient positioning (Mandibular lateral and canine). **B** Diagram of the positioning. **C** Plan view of the positioning. **D** Resultant radiograph with the main radiographic features indicated.

Mandibular premolars

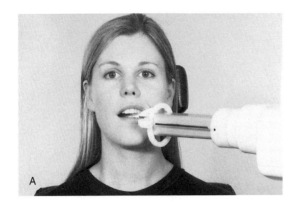

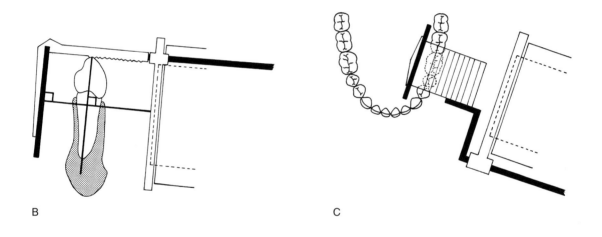

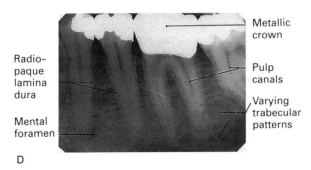

Fig. 8.11A Patient positioning (Mandibular premolars). **B** Diagram of the positioning. **C** Plan view of the positioning. **D** Resultant radiograph with the main radiographic features indicated.

Mandibular molars

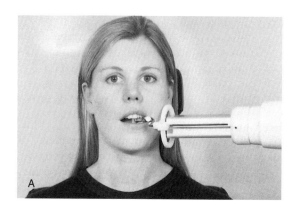

A

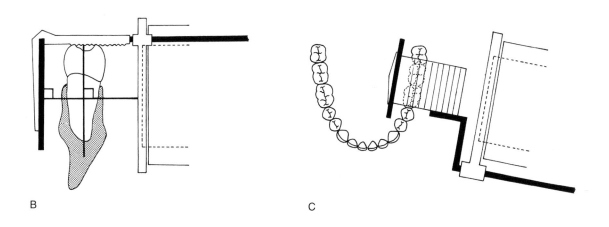

B

C

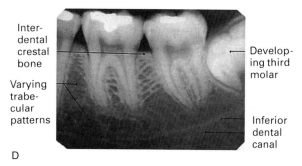

Inter-
dental
crestal
bone

Develop-
ing third
molar

Varying
trabe-
cular
patterns

Inferior
dental
canal

D

Fig. 8.12A Patient positioning (Mandibular molars). **B** Diagram of the positioning. **C** Plan view of the positioning.
D Resultant radiograph with the main radiographic features indicated.

Bisected angle technique

Theory

The theoretical basis of the bisected angle technique is shown in Figure 8.13 and can be summarized as follows:

1. The film packet is placed as close to the tooth under investigation as possible without bending the packet.
2. The angle formed between the long axis of the tooth and the long axis of the film packet is assessed and mentally bisected.
3. The X-ray tubehead is positioned at right angles to this bisecting line with the central ray of the X-ray beam aimed through the tooth apex.
4. Using the geometrical principle of similar triangles, the actual length of the tooth in the mouth will be equal to the length of the image of the tooth on the film.

Vertical angulation of the X-ray tubehead

The angle formed by continuing the line of the central ray until it meets the occlusal plane determines the *vertical angulation* of the X-ray beam to the occlusal plane (see Fig. 8.13).

Note: These vertical angles are often quoted but inevitably they are only approximate. Patient differences including head position, and individual tooth position and inclination mean that each positioning should be assessed independently. The vertical angulations suggested should be taken only as a general guide.

Horizontal angulation of the X-ray tubehead

In the horizontal plane, the central ray should be aimed through the interproximal contact areas, to avoid overlapping the teeth. The *horizontal angulation* is therefore determined by the shape of the arch and the position of the teeth (see Fig. 8.14).

Positioning techniques

The bisected angle technique can be performed either by using a film holder to support the film packet in the patient's mouth or by asking the patient to support the film packet **gently** using either an index finger or thumb. Using a film holder is the recommended technique to avoid irradiating the patient's fingers. However, using the finger is still widely used and both techniques are described and illustrated.

Using film holders

Various film holders are available, a selection of which are shown in Figure 8.15. The Rinn Bisected Angle Instruments (BAI) closely resemble the paralleling technique holders and consist of the same three basic components — film-holding

Central ray of the
X-ray beam aimed through
the tooth apex

Long axis of the tooth
Bisecting line

Long axis of the filr

2–3 mm of film
visible beyond the
incisal edge

Vertical angulation

Fig. 8.13 Theoretical basis of the bisected angle technique. The angle between the long axes of the tooth and film is bisected and X-ray beam aimed at right angles to this line, through the apex of the tooth. With this geometrical arrangement, the length of the tooth in the mouth is equal to the length of the image of the tooth on the film, but, as shown, the periodontal bone levels will not be represented accurately.

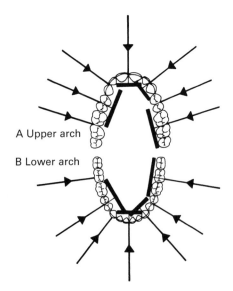

A Upper arch

B Lower arch

Fig. 8.14 Diagram of **A** the upper arch and **B** the lower arch. The various horizontal angulations of the X-ray beam are shown.

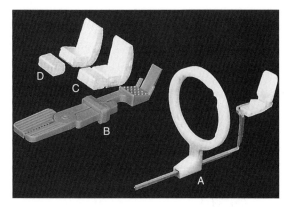

Fig. 8.15 A selection of film packet holders for the bisected angle technique. **A** The Rinn bisected angle instrument (BAI). **B** The Emmenix® film holder. **C** The Rinn Greene Stabe® bite block. **D** The Rinn Greene Stabe® bite block reduced in size for easier positioning and for use in children.

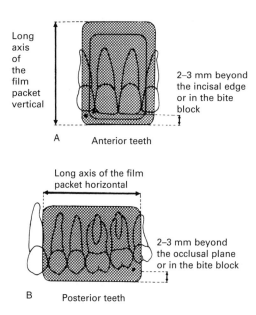

Fig. 8.16 Diagrams showing the general requirements of the film packet position for **A** anterior and **B** posterior teeth.

mechanism, bite block and an X-ray beam-aiming device — but the film is not held parallel to the teeth. The more simple holders and the disposable bite blocks hold the film packet in the desired position but the X-ray tubehead then has to be aligned independently. In summary:

1. The film packet is pushed securely into the chosen holder. Either a large or small size of film packet is used so that the particular tooth being examined is in the middle of the film, as shown in Figure 8.16 with the white surface of the film packet facing the X-ray tubehead and with the film orientation dot opposite the crown.

2. The X-ray tubehead is positioned using the beam-aiming device if available OR the operator has to assess the *vertical* and *horizontal angulations* and then position the tubehead independently.

3. The exposure is made.

Using the patient's finger

1. The appropriate sized film packet is positioned and orientated in the mouth as shown in Figure 8.16 with about 2 mm extending beyond the incisal or occlusal edges, to ensure that all of the tooth will appear on the film. The patient is then asked to gently support the film packet using either an index finger or thumb.

2. The operator then assesses the *vertical* and *horizontal angulations* and positions the tubehead independently. The effects of incorrect tubehead position are shown in Figure 8.17.

3. The exposure is made.

The specific positioning for different areas of the mouth, using both simple holders and the patient's finger to support the film packet, is shown in Figures 8.18–8.25.

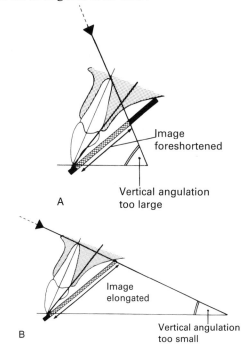

Fig. 8.17 Diagrams showing the effects of incorrect vertical tubehead positioning. **A** Foreshortening of the image. **B** Elongation of the image.

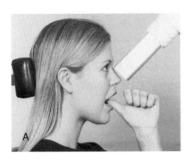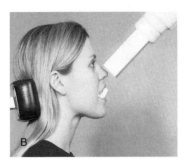

Maxillary central incisors

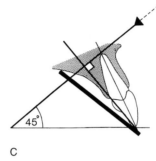

C

Fig. 8.18 Patient positioning with the patient **A** supporting the film packet with the ball of the left thumb and **B** using the Rinn Greene Stabe® bite block. **C** Diagram of the relative positions of film, tooth and X-ray beam.

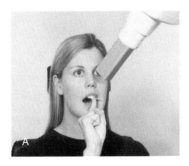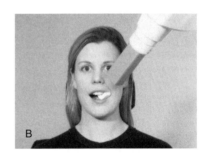

Maxillary canine

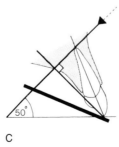

C

Fig. 8.19 Patient positioning with the patient **A** supporting the film packet with the ball of the right index finger and **B** using the Rinn Greene Stabe® bite block. **C** Diagram of the relative positions of film, tooth and X-ray beam.

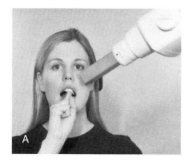
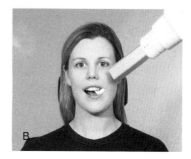

Maxillary premolars

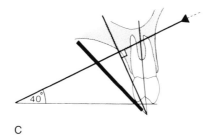

C

Fig. 8.20 Patient positioning with the patient **A** supporting the film packet and **B** using the Rinn Greene Stabe® bite block. **C** Diagram of the relative positions of film, tooth and X-ray beam.

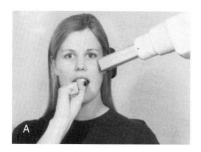
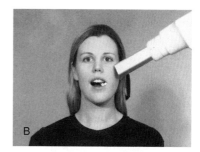

Maxillary molars

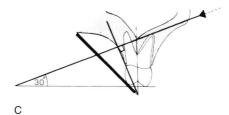

C

Fig. 8.21 Patient positioning with the patient **A** supporting the film packet and **B** using the Rinn Greene Stabe® bite block. **C** Diagram of the relative positions of film, tooth and X-ray beam.

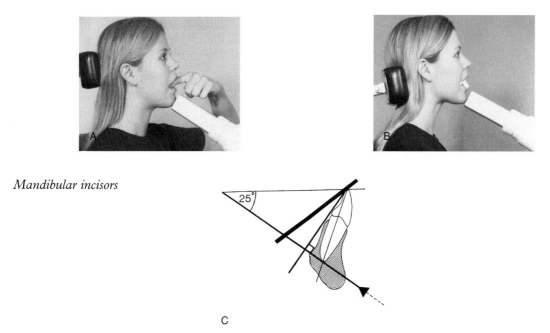

Mandibular incisors

C

Fig. 8.22 Patient positioning with **A** the patient's index finger on the upper edge of the film packet, supporting and depressing it into the floor of the mouth and **B** using the Rinn Greene Stabe® bite block. **C** Diagram of the relative positions of film, tooth and X-ray beam.

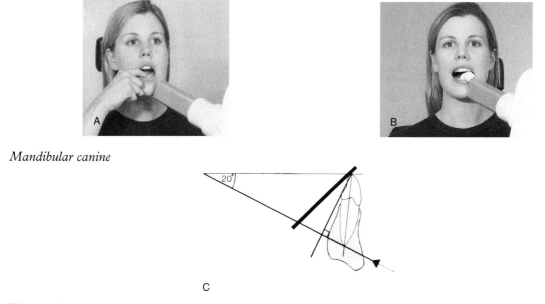

Mandibular canine

C

Fig. 8.23 Patient positioning with the patient **A** supporting and depressing the upper edge of the film packet and **B** using the Rinn Greene Stabe® bite block. **C** Diagram of the relative positions of film, tooth and X-ray beam.

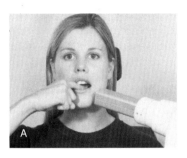
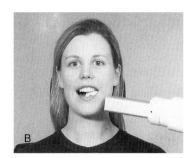

Mandibular premolars

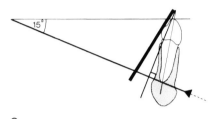

C

Fig. 8.24 Patient positioning with the patient **A** supporting the film packet and **B** using the Rinn Greene Stabe® bite block. **C** Diagram of the relative positions of film, tooth and X-ray beam.

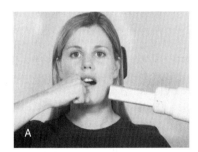
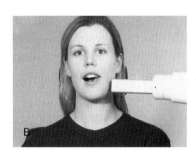

Mandibular molars

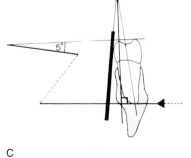

C

Fig. 8.25 Patient positioning with the patient **A** supporting the film packet and **B** using the Rinn Greene Stabe® bite block. **C** Diagram of the relative positions of film, tooth and X-ray beam.

Full-mouth survey

This terminology is used to describe a collection of periapical radiographs showing the full dentition. Not every tooth is radiographed individually, but enough films are taken to include all the teeth.

Comparison of the paralleling and bisected angle techniques

The advantages and disadvantages of the two techniques can be summarized as follows:

Advantages of the paralleling technique

- Geometrically accurate images are produced with little magnification.
- The shadow of the zygomatic buttress appears **above** the apices of the molar teeth.
- The periodontal bone levels are well represented.
- The periapical tissues are accurately shown with minimal foreshortening or elongation.
- The crowns of the teeth are well shown enabling the detection of approximal caries.
- The horizontal and vertical angulations of the X-ray tubehead are automatically determined by the positioning devices if placed correctly.
- The X-ray beam is aimed accurately at the centre of the film — all areas of the film are irradiated and there is no *coning off* or *cone cutting*.
- Reproducible radiographs are possible at different visits and with different operators.
- The relative positions of the film packet, teeth and X-ray beam are always maintained, irrespective of the position of the patient's head. This is useful for some patients with disabilities.

Disadvantages of the paralleling technique

- Positioning of the film packet can be very uncomfortable for the patient, particularly for posterior teeth, often causing gagging.
- Positioning the holders within the mouth can be difficult for inexperienced operators.
- The anatomy of the mouth sometimes makes the technique impossible, e.g. a shallow, flat palate.

- The apices of the teeth can sometimes appear very near the edge of the film.
- Positioning the holders in the lower third molar regions can be very difficult.
- The technique cannot be performed satisfactorily using a short focal spot to skin distance (i.e. a short spacer cone) because of the resultant magnification.
- The holders need to be autoclavable or disposable.

Advantages of the bisected angle technique

- Positioning of the film packet is reasonably comfortable for the patient in all areas of the mouth.
- Positioning is relatively simple and quick.
- If all angulations are assessed correctly, the image of the tooth will be the same length as the tooth itself and should be *adequate* (but not ideal) for most diagnostic purposes.

Disadvantages of the bisected angle technique

- The many variables involved in the technique often result in the image being badly distorted.
- Incorrect vertical angulation will result in foreshortening or elongation of the image.
- The periodontal bone levels are poorly shown.
- The shadow of the zygomatic buttress frequently overlies the roots of the upper molars.
- The horizontal and vertical angles have to be assessed for every patient and considerable skill is required.
- It is not possible to obtain reproducible views.
- *Coning off* or *cone cutting* may result if the central ray is not aimed at the centre of the film, particularly if using rectangular collimation.
- Incorrect horizontal angulation will result in overlapping of the crowns and roots.
- The crowns of the teeth are often distorted, thus preventing the detection of approximal caries.
- The buccal roots of the maxillary premolars and molars are foreshortened.

A visual comparison between the two techniques, showing how dramatic the variation in image quality and reproductibility can be, is shown in Figures 8.26 and 8.27.

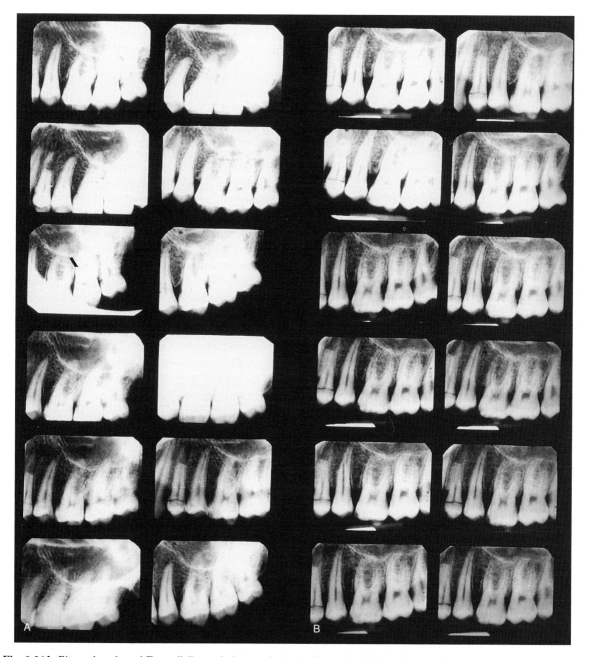

Fig. 8.26A Bisected angle and **B** paralleling technique periapical radiographs of ⌞6, on the *same* phantom head, taken by 12 *different* experienced operators. The obvious reproducibility and accurate imaging show why the paralleling technique should be regarded as the technique of choice.

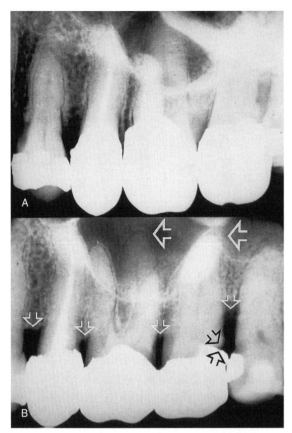

Fig. 8.27A Bisected angle and **B** paralleling technique periapicals of the /45678 taken on the *same* patient, by the *same* operator, on the *same* day. Note the difference in the periodontal bone levels (small white open arrows), the restoration in /7 (black open arrows) and the apical tissues /67 (large white open arrows).

Conclusion

The diagnostic advantages of the accurate, reproducible images produced by the paralleling technique using film holders and beam-aiming devices ensure that this technique should be regarded as the technique of choice for periapical radiography. Their use is recommended by the NRPB/RCR in their document *Guidelines on Radiology Standards in Primary Dental Care* and in the new 2001 *Guidance Notes* (see Ch. 6).

Positioning difficulties often encountered in periapical radiography

Placing the film packet intraorally in the *textbook-described* positions is not always possible. The radiographic techniques described earlier often need to be modified. The main difficulties encountered involve:

* Mandibular third molars
* Gagging
* Endodontics
* Edentulous alveolar ridges
* Children
* Patients with disabilities (see Ch. 7).

Problems posed by mandibular third molars

The main difficulty is placement of the film packet sufficiently posteriorly to record the entire third mandibular molar (particularly when it is horizontally impacted) **and** the surrounding tissues, including the inferior dental canal (see Fig. 8.28).

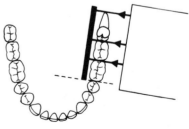

Fig. 8.28 Diagrams showing the ideal film packet position for mandibular third molars to ensure the tooth and apical tissues are recorded.

Possible solutions

These include:

• Using specially designed or adapted holders as shown in Figure 8.29 to hold and position the film packet in the mouth, as follows:

1. The holder is clipped securely on to the top edge of the film packet.

2. With the mouth open, the film packet is positioned gently in the lingual sulcus as far posteriorly as possible.

3. The patient is asked to close the mouth (so relaxing the tissues of the floor of the mouth) and at the same time the film packet is eased further back into the mouth, if required, until its front edge is opposite the mesial surface of the mandibular first molar.

4. The patient is asked to bite on the holder and to support it in position.

5. The X-ray tubehead is positioned at right angles to the third molar and the film packet and centred 1 cm up from the lower border of the mandible, on a vertical line dropped from the outer corner of the eye (see Fig. 8.29).

• Taking two radiographs of the third molar using two different horizontal tubehead angulations, as follows:

1. The film packet is positioned as posteriorly as possible (using the technique described with the holders).

2. The X-ray tubehead is aimed with the *ideal* horizontal angulation so the X-ray beam passes between the second and third molars. (With horizontally impacted third molars, the apex may not be recorded using this positioning, as shown in Figure 8.30.)

3. A *second* film packet is placed in the same position as before, but the X-ray tubehead is

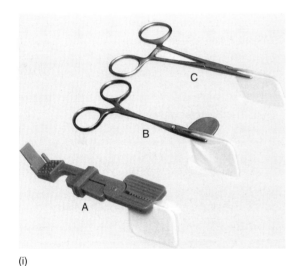

(i)

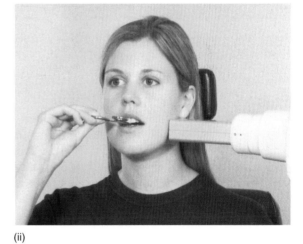

(ii)

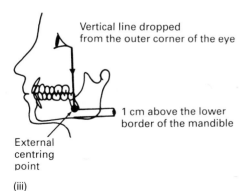

Vertical line dropped
from the outer corner of the eye

1 cm above the lower
border of the mandible

External
centring
point

(iii)

Fig. 8.29(i) A selection of film packet holders for mandibular third molars: **A** Emmenix® film holder. **B** Worth film holder and **C** a conventional pair of artery forceps. **(ii)** Patient positioning—having closed the mouth, the patient is stabilizing the film packet holder with a hand. **(iii)** Diagram indicating the external centring point for the X-ray beam.

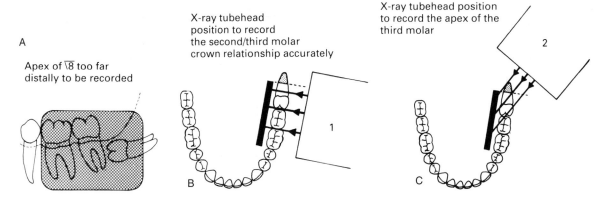

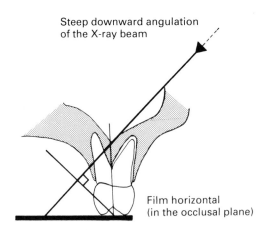

Fig. 8.30 The problem of the horizontal third molar. **A** Side view showing the often achievable film packet position. **B** Plan view showing X-ray tubehead position 1. **C** Plan view showing X-ray tubehead position 2.

positioned further posteriorly aiming forwards to project the apex of the third molar on to the film. (With this positioning, the crowns of the second and third molars will be overlapped, as shown in Figure 8.30.)

Note: The vertical angulation of the X-ray tubehead is the same for both projections.

Problems of gagging

The gag reflex is particularly strong in some patients. This makes the placement of the film packet in the desired position particularly difficult, especially in the upper and lower molar regions.

Possible solutions

These include:

- Patient sucking a local anaesthetic lozenge before attempting to position the film packet
- Asking the patient to concentrate on breathing deeply while the film packet is in the mouth
- Placing the film packet flat in the mouth (in the occlusal plane) so it does not touch the

palate, and applying the principles of the bisected angle technique — the long axes of the tooth and film packet are assessed and the X-ray tubehead's position modified accordingly, as shown in Figure 8.31.

Fig. 8.31 Diagram showing the relative position of the X-ray beam to the maxillary molar and film, when the film is placed in the occlusal plane. **Note**: The length of the image of the tooth on the radiograph should again equal the length of the tooth in the mouth. However, there will be considerable distortion of the surrounding tissues.

Problems encountered during endodontics

The main difficulties involve:

- Film packet placement and stabilization when endodontic instruments, rubber dam and rubber dam clamps are in position
- Identification and separation of root canals
- Assessing root canal lengths from foreshortened or elongated radiographs.

Possible solutions

These include:

- The problem of film packet placement and stabilization can be solved by:
  — Using a simple film packet holder such as the Rinn Eezee-Grip®, as shown in Figure 8.32. This is positioned in the mouth and then held in place by the patient.
  — Using one of the special endodontic film holders that have been developed. These incorporate a small basket in the bite platform area, to accommodate the handles of the endodontic instruments, while still allowing the film packet and the tooth to be parallel. (See Fig. 8.33.)

- The problem of identifying and separating the root canals can be solved by taking at least two radiographs, using different horizontal X-ray tubehead positions, as shown in Figure 8.34.
- The problems of assessing root canal length can be solved by:
  — Taking an accurate paralleling technique periapical preoperatively and measuring the lengths of the root(s) directly from the radiograph before beginning the endodontic treatment. The amount of distortion on subsequent films can then be assessed.
  — Calculating mathematically the actual length of a root canal from a distorted bisected angle technique periapical taken with the diagnostic instrument within the root canal at the clinically assessed apical *stop*.

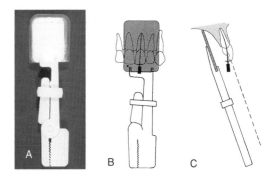

Fig. 8.32A The Rinn Eezee–Grip® film holder. **B** and **C** Diagrams showing its use in endodontics. (**Note:** Rubber dam not shown.)

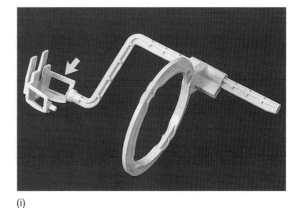

(i)

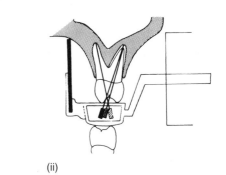

(ii)

Fig. 8.33 (i) A specially designed film packet holder (Rinn Endoray®) for use during endodontics, incorporating a basket (arrowed) to accommodate the handles of the endodontic instruments and a beam-aiming device. **(ii)** Diagram of the holder in place.

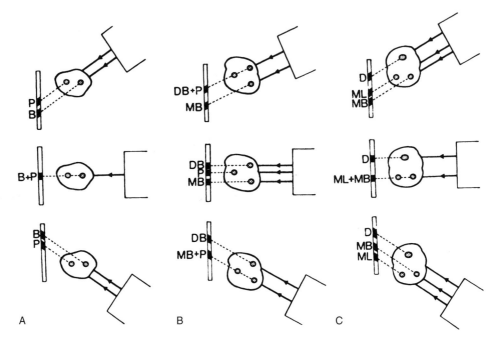

Fig. 8.34 Diagrams showing the effect of different horizontal X-ray tubehead positions on root separation for **A** maxillary premolars, **B** maxillary first molars and **C** mandibular first molars. (The images of the canals are designated: P = palatal, B = buccal, MB = mesiobuccal, DB = distobuccal, ML = mesiolingual and D = distal.)

The calculation is done as follows (see Fig. 8.35):

1. Measure:
   a. The *radiographic tooth length*
   b. The *radiographic instrument length*
   c. The *actual instrument length*

2. Substitute the measurements into the formula:

$$\text{Actual tooth length} = \frac{\text{Radiographic tooth length} \times \text{Actual instrument length}}{\text{Radiographic instrument length}}$$

3. Calculate the *actual tooth length* and adjust the working length of the instrument as necessary.

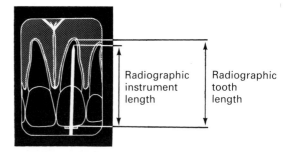

Fig. 8.35 Diagram showing the required radiographic measurements in endodontics to calculate the actual tooth length.

Problems of the edentulous ridge

The main difficulty in the edentulous and partially dentate patient is again film packet placement.

Possible solutions

These include:

• In edentulous patients, the lack of height in the palate, or loss of lingual sulcus depth, contraindicates the paralleling technique and all periapical radiographs should be taken using a modified bisected angle technique. The long axes of the film packet and the alveolar ridge are assessed and the X-ray tubehead position adjusted accordingly as shown in Figure 8.36.

• In partially dentate patients, the paralleling technique can usually be used. If the edentulous area causes the film packet holder to be displaced, the deficiency can be built up by using cottonwool rolls, as shown in Figure 8.37.

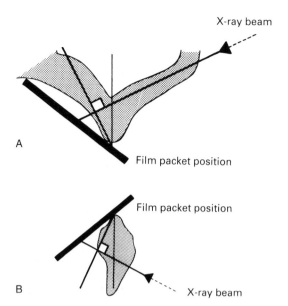

Fig. 8.36 Diagrams showing the relative position of the film packet and X-ray beam. **A** For the molar region of an edentulous maxillary ridge. **B** For the molar region of an edentulous mandibular ridge.

Problems encountered in children

Once again the main technical problem (as opposed to management problems) encountered in children is the size of their mouths and the difficulty in placing the film packet intraorally. The paralleling technique is not possible in very small children, but can often be used (and is recommended) anteriorly, for investigating traumatized permanent incisors. The reproducibility afforded by this technique is invaluable for future comparative purposes.

A modified bisected angle technique is possible in most children, with the film placed flat in the mouth (in the occlusal plane) and the position of the X-ray tubehead adjusted accordingly, as shown in Figure 8.38.

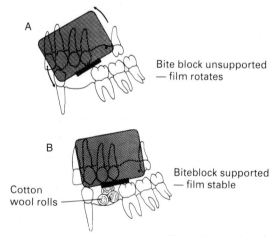

Fig. 8.37 Diagrams showing **A** the effect on the position of the film packet and holder created by an edentulous area, and **B** how the problem can be solved using cottonwool rolls to rebuild the edentulous area, thus supporting the bite block.

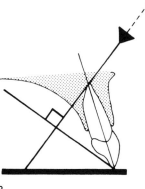

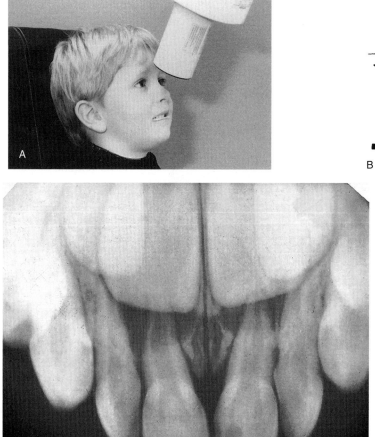

Fig. 8.38A Positioning for a child's maxillary incisors. **B** Diagram showing the relative positions of the film packet, in the occlusal plane, and the X-ray beam. **C** Resultant radiograph.

Footnote

Periapical radiography is not always as straightforward in practice as it appears in theory. Although the paralleling technique should be regarded as the technique of choice, it is not always possible. However, a knowledge of the theoretical requirements of imaging enables the clinician to modify the available techniques to suit individual needs of patients.

9 Bitewing radiography

Bitewing radiographs take their name from the original technique which required the patient to *bite* on a small *wing* attached to an intraoral film packet (see Fig. 9.1). Modern film holders, as shown later, have eliminated the need for the wing (now termed a *tab*), but the terminology and clinical indications have remained the same. An individual film is designed to show the crowns of the premolar and molar teeth on one side of the jaws.

Main indications

The main clinical indications include:

- Detection of dental caries
- Monitoring the progression of dental caries
- Assessment of existing restorations
- Assessment of the periodontal status.

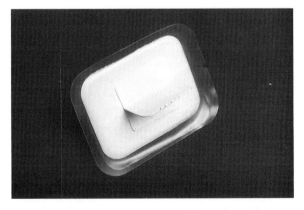

Fig. 9.1 An intraoral barrier-wrapped film packet with a *wing* or *tab* attached.

Ideal technique requirements

These include:

- The *tab* or bite-platform should be positioned on the middle of the film packet and parallel to the upper and lower edges of the film packet.
- The film packet should be positioned with its long axis horizontally for a *horizontal bitewing* or vertically for a *vertical bitewing* (Fig. 9.2).
- The posterior teeth and the film packet should be in contact or as close together as possible.
- The posterior teeth and the film packet should be parallel — the shape of the dental arch may necessitate two separate film positions to achieve this requirement for the premolars and the molars (Fig. 9.3).
- In the horizontal plane, the X-ray tubehead should be aimed so that the beam meets the teeth and the film packet at right angles, and passes directly through **all** the contact areas (Fig. 9.3).
- In the vertical plane, the X-ray tubehead should be aimed downwards (approximately 5°–8° to the horizontal) to compensate for the upwardly rising curve of Monson (Fig. 9.4).
- The positioning should be reproducible.

Positioning techniques

There are two main techniques available:

- Using a tab attached to the film packet and aligning the X-ray tubehead by eye
- Using a film packet holder with beam-aiming device to facilitate the positioning and alignment of the X-ray tubehead.

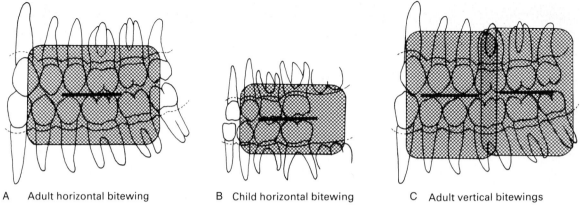

A   Adult horizontal bitewing   B   Child horizontal bitewing   C   Adult vertical bitewings

Fig. 9.2 Diagrams showing the ideal film packet position for different types of bitewings.

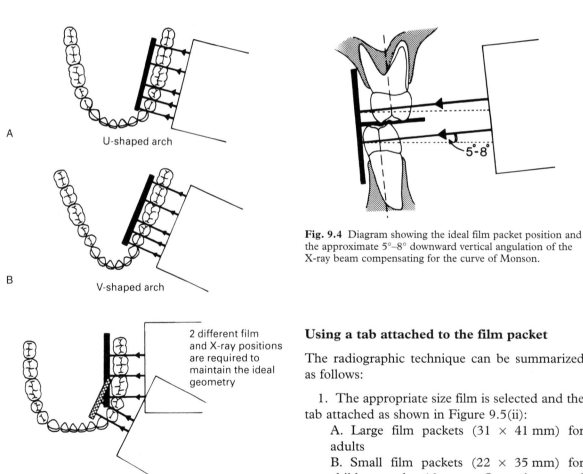

A   U-shaped arch

B   V-shaped arch

C   Square arch

2 different film and X-ray positions are required to maintain the ideal geometry

Fig. 9.3 Diagrams showing the ideal film packet and X-ray tube positions for bitewing radiography for different dental arch shapes.

5–8°

Fig. 9.4 Diagram showing the ideal film packet position and the approximate 5°–8° downward vertical angulation of the X-ray beam compensating for the curve of Monson.

Using a tab attached to the film packet

The radiographic technique can be summarized as follows:

1. The appropriate size film is selected and the tab attached as shown in Figure 9.5(ii):

A. Large film packets (31 × 41 mm) for adults

B. Small film packets (22 × 35 mm) for children under 12 years. Once the second permanent molars have erupted the adult size film is required

C. Occasionally a longer film packet (53 × 26 mm) is used for adults.

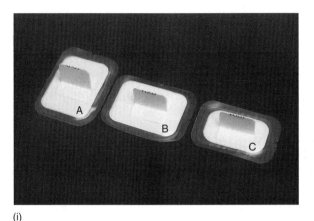

(i)

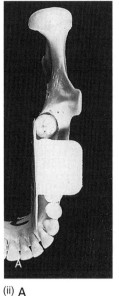

(ii) A

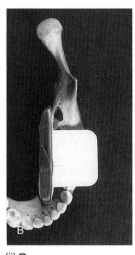

(ii) B

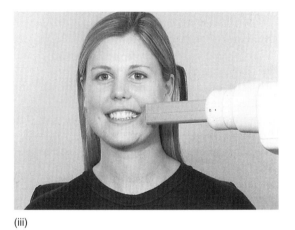

(iii)

Fig. 9.5 (i) Film packets with tabs attached suitable for **A** adult vertical bitewings, **B** adult horizontal bitewings and **C** child's horizontal bitewings. **(ii)** The ideal bitewing and film packet position in relation to the teeth for **A** an adult and **B** a child. **(iii)** Patient and X-ray tubehead positioning for a left bitewing.

2. The patient is positioned with the head supported and with the occlusal plane horizontal.

3. The shape of the dental arch and the number of films required are assessed.

4. The operator holds the tab between thumb and forefinger and inserts the film packet into the lingual sulcus opposite the posterior teeth.

5. The anterior edge of the film packet should be positioned opposite the distal aspect of the lower canine — in this position, the posterior edge of the film packet extends usually just beyond the mesial aspect of the lower third molar.

6. The tab is placed on to the occlusal surfaces of the lower teeth.

7. The patient is asked to close the teeth firmly together on to the tab.

8. As the patient closes the teeth, the operator pulls the tab firmly between the teeth to ensure that the film packet and the teeth are in contact.

9. The operator releases the tab.

10. The X-ray beam is aimed directly through the contact areas, at right angles to the teeth and the film packet, with an approximate 5°–8° downward vertical angulation.

11. The exposure is made.

12. The procedure is repeated for the premolar teeth, if required, with a new film packet and X-ray tubehead position.

Note: When positioning the X-ray tubehead, after the patient has closed the mouth, the film can no longer be seen. To ensure that the anterior part of the film is exposed and to avoid *coning off* or *cone cutting*, a simple guide to remember is that the front edge of the open-ended spacer cone should be positioned adjacent to the corner of the mouth.

Advantages

- Simple
- Inexpensive
- The tabs are disposable, so no extra cross-infection control procedures required
- Can be used easily in children.

Disadvantages

- Arbitrary, operator-dependent assessment of horizontal and vertical angulations of the X-ray tubehead
- Radiographs not accurately reproducible, so not suitable for monitoring the progression of caries.
- *Coning off* or *cone cutting* of anterior part of film is common
- The tongue can easily displace the film packet.

Using simple film packet holders

Several simple film holders have been produced, a selection of which is shown in Figure 9.6. They can eliminate many of the disadvantages of the arbitrary tab method. As in periapical radiography, the choice of holder is a matter of personal preference. Holders vary in cost and design but essentially consist of three basic components:

- A mechanism for holding the film packet parallel to the teeth
- A bite-platform that replaces the wing
- An X-ray beam-aiming device.

The position of the Hawe–Neos Kwikbite holders, favoured by the author, in relation to the teeth and in clinical use is illustrated in Figure 9.7.

Advantages

- Simple
- Film packet held firmly in position and cannot be displaced by the tongue
- Position of X-ray tubehead determined by the holder, thus is less operator-dependent, ensuring that the X-ray beam is always at right angles to the film packet
- Avoids *coning off* or *cone cutting* of anterior part of film
- Holders are autoclavable or disposable.

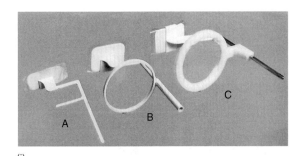

(i)

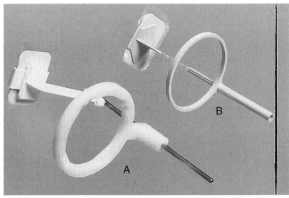

(ii)

Fig. 9.6 A selection of bitewing film packet holders **(i)** suitable for *horizontal bitewings*: *A* Hawe–Neos Kwikbite with simple beam-indicating rod; **B** Hawe–Neos Kwikbite with circular beam-aiming device; **C** Rinn bitewing holder; and **(ii)** suitable for *vertical* bitewings: **A** Rinn holder; **B** Hawe–Neos holder.

Disadvantages

- Position of the holder in the mouth is operator-dependent, therefore not 100% reproducible, so still not ideal for monitoring progression of caries
- Positioning of the film holder can be uncomfortable for the patient
- Some holders are relatively expensive
- Holders not usually suitable for children.

Conclusion

Traditional bitewing techniques, using detachable tabs, although simple to perform and still used widely are operator-dependent and inaccurate. The more accurate techniques using film holders and beam-aiming devices, which are less dependent on subjective assessments, are strongly recommended.

Whichever radiographic technique is used, the resultant radiographs and the anatomical structures they show are very similar — it is their accuracy that varies. Examples are shown in Figures 9.8–9.10.

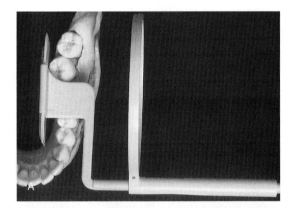
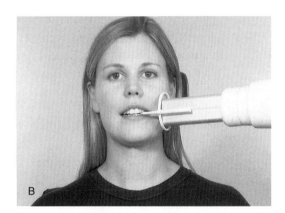
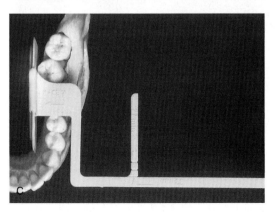
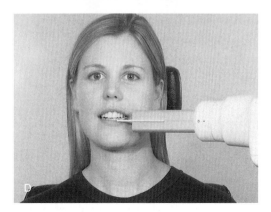

Fig. 9.7A Position of the horizontal Hawe–Neos Kwikbite holder (with circular beam-aiming device) in relation to the teeth. **B** In clinical use. **C** Position of the Hawe–Neos simple Kwikbite holder in relation to the teeth. **D** In clinical use.

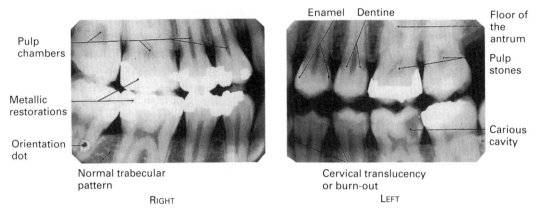

Fig. 9.8 Examples of typical RIGHT and LEFT horizontal adult bitewing radiographs, suitable for the assessment of caries and restorations, with the main radiographic features indicated.

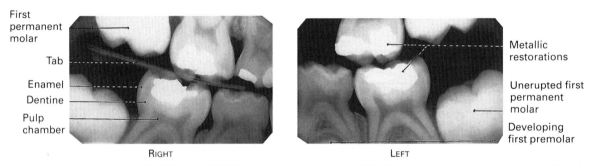

Fig. 9.9 Examples of typical RIGHT and LEFT bitewing radiographs of a child with the main radiographic features indicated.

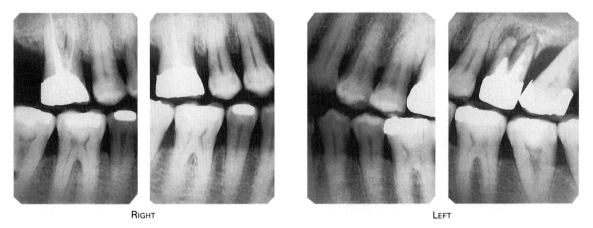

Fig. 9.10 Example of typical RIGHT and LEFT vertical adult bitewing radiographs. Note that two films are used on each side to image both the premolars and molars.

Ideal exposure factors

The clinical reasons for taking a bitewing radiograph should determine the exposure factors that are used, for example:

- *Assessment of caries and restorations* — films should be well exposed and show good contrast to allow differentiation between enamel and dentine and to allow the enamel — dentine junction (EDJ) to be seen.
- *Assessment of periodontal status* — films should be under-exposed to avoid *burn-out* of the thin alveolar crestal bone.

The effect of varying the exposure factors, including what happens to the EDJ and the alveolar crestal bone is shown in Figure 9.11.

To satisfy **both** ideal exposure requirements, two sets of bitewings would be required routinely. In practice, a typical pair of bitewings often involves a compromise with regard to the exposure factors. In this way, the radiation dose to the patient is kept to a minimum but the resultant radiographs may not be ideal for **all** diagnostic purposes. This is considered further in Chapters 18 and 20.

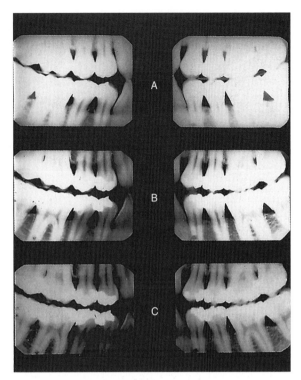

Fig. 9.11 Three pairs of bitewing radiographs taken on the same patient but with varying exposure factors. **A** Reduced exposure. **B** Normal exposure. **C** Increased exposure. Note the increasing contrast between enamel and dentine as the exposure increases, but also the increasing amount of *burn-out* of the alveolar crestal bone and cervical portions of the teeth.

10 Occlusal radiography

Occlusal radiography is defined as those intraoral radiographic techniques taken using a dental X-ray set where the film packet (5.7 × 7.6 cm) or a small intraoral cassette is placed in the occlusal plane.

Terminology and classification

The terminology used in occlusal radiography is very confusing. The British Standards Glossary of Dental Terms (BS 4492: 1983) is inadequate in defining the various occlusal projections and in differentiating between them. The result is that there is still little uniformity in terminology among different publications and teaching institutions.

The terminology used here is based broadly on the British Standards terms, but they have been modified in an attempt to make them more explicit, straightforward and practical so that often the name of the view indicates how it is taken. The terms used in the British Standards Glossary are included in brackets.

Maxillary occlusal projections

- *Upper standard occlusal* (standard occlusal)
- *Upper oblique occlusal* (oblique occlusal)
- *Vertex occlusal* (vertex occlusal).

Mandibular occlusal projections

- *Lower 90° occlusal* (true occlusal)
- *Lower 45° occlusal* (standard occlusal)
- *Lower oblique occlusal* (oblique occlusal).

Upper standard occlusal

This projection shows the anterior part of the maxilla and the upper anterior teeth.

Main clinical indications

The main clinical indications include:

- Periapical assessment of the upper anterior teeth, especially in children but also in adults unable to tolerate periapical films
- Detecting the presence of unerupted canines, supernumeraries and odontomes
- As the midline view, when using the parallax method for determining the bucco/palatal position of unerupted canines
- Evaluation of the size and extent of lesions such as cysts or tumours in the anterior maxilla
- Assessment of fractures of the anterior teeth and alveolar bone. It is especially useful in children following trauma because film placement is straightforward.

Technique and positioning

The technique can be summarized as follows:

1. The patient is seated with the head supported and with the occlusal plane horizontal and parallel to the floor and is asked to support a protective thyroid shield.

2. The film packet, with the white (pebbly) surface facing uppermost, is placed flat into the mouth on to the occlusal surfaces of the lower teeth. The patient is asked to bite together gently. The film packet is placed centrally in the mouth with its long axis crossways in adults and anteroposteriorly in children.

3. The X-ray tubehead is positioned above the patient in the midline, aiming downwards through the bridge of the nose at an angle of 65°–70° to the film packet (see Fig. 10.1).

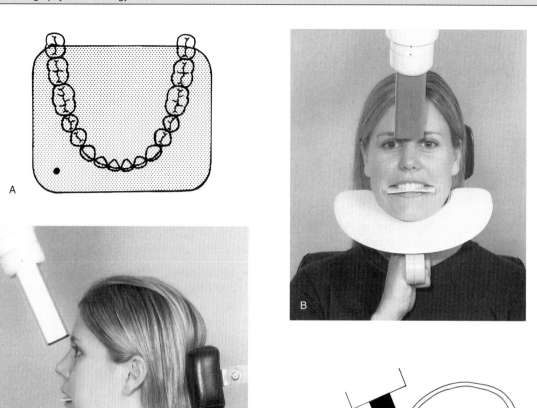

Fig. 10.1A Diagram showing the position of the film packet in relation to the lower arch. **B** Positioning from the front; note the use of the protective thyroid shield. **C** Positioning from the side. **D** Diagram showing the positioning from the side.

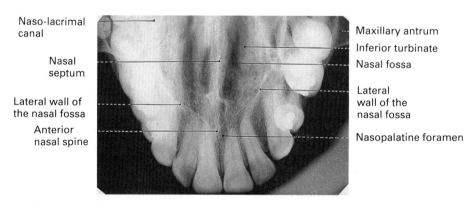

Fig. 10.2 An example of an upper standard occlusal radiograph with the main radiographic features indicated.

Upper oblique occlusal

This projection shows the posterior part of the maxilla and the upper posterior teeth on one side.

Main clinical indications

- Periapical assessment of the upper posterior teeth, especially in adults unable to tolerate periapical films
- Evaluation of the size and extent of lesions such as cysts, tumours or osteodystrophies affecting the posterior maxilla
- Assessment of the condition of the antral floor
- As an aid to determining the position of roots displaced inadvertently into the antrum during attempted extraction of upper posterior teeth
- Assessment of fractures of the posterior teeth and associated alveolar bone including the tuberosity.

Technique and positioning

1. The patient is seated with the head supported and with the occlusal plane horizontal and parallel to the floor.

2. The film packet, with the white (pebbly) surface facing uppermost, is inserted into the mouth on to the occlusal surfaces of the lower teeth, with its long axis anteroposteriorly. It is placed to the side of the mouth under investigation, and the patient is asked to bite together gently.

3. The X-ray tubehead is positioned to the side of the patient's face, aiming downwards through the cheek at an angle of 65°–70° to the film, centring on the region of interest (see Fig. 10.3).

Note: If the X-ray tubehead is positioned too far posteriorly, the shadow cast by the body of the zygoma will obscure the posterior teeth.

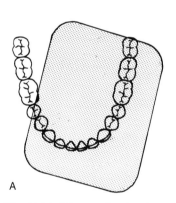
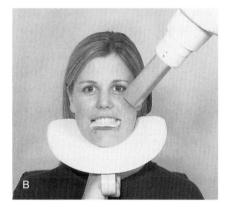
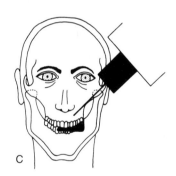

A   B   C

Fig. 10.3A Diagram showing the position of the film packet in relation to the lower arch for a LEFT upper oblique occlusal. **B** Positioning for the LEFT upper oblique occlusal from the front; note the use of the protective thyroid shield. **C** Diagram showing the positioning from the front.

Resultant radiograph

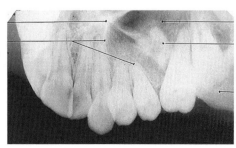

Floor of the nasal fossa

Anterior wall and floor of the antrum

Maxillary antrum

Retained root of /6

Zygoma

Fig. 10.4 An example of an upper left oblique occlusal radiograph with the main radiographic features indicated.

Vertex occlusal

This projection shows a plan view of the tooth-bearing portion of the maxilla from above. To obtain this view the X-ray beam has to pass through a considerable amount of tissue, delivering a large dose of radiation to the patient. An intraoral *cassette* containing intensifying screens is used for this projection to reduce the dose.

Main clinical indication

- Assessment of the bucco/palatal position of unerupted canines.

Technique and positioning

The technique can be summarized as follows:

1. The patient is seated with the head supported and with the occlusal plane horizontal and parallel to the floor.

2. The cassette is placed inside a small plastic bag to prevent salivary contamination and cross-infection.

3. It is then inserted into the mouth on to the occlusal surfaces of the lower teeth, with its long axis anteroposteriorly and the patient is asked to bite on to it.

4. The X-ray tubehead is positioned above the patient, in the midline, aiming downwards through the vertex of the skull. The main beam is therefore aimed approximately down the long axis of the root canals of the upper incisor teeth (see Fig. 10.5).

Disadvantages

The vertex occlusal projection is not often used because it has several drawbacks and disadvantages:

- There is a lack of detail and contrast on the film because of the intensifying screens, the mass of tissue the X-ray beam has to penetrate and the consequent scatter.
- The primary X-ray beam may be in direct line with the reproductive organs.
- A relatively long exposure time is needed (about 1 second) despite the use of intensifying screens.
- There is direct radiation to the pituitary gland and the lens of the eye.
- If the X-ray beam is positioned too far anteriorly, superimposition of the shadow of the frontal bones may obscure the anterior part of the maxilla.

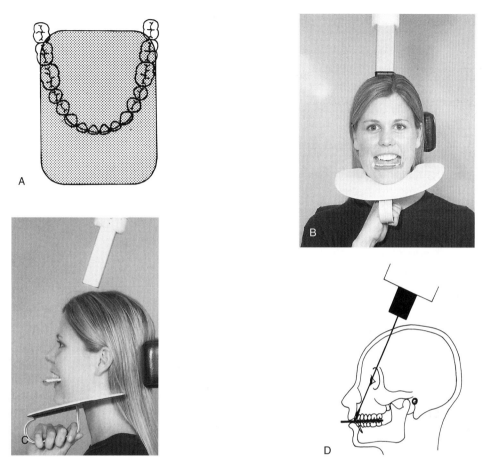

Fig. 10.5A Diagram showing the position of the cassette in relation to the lower arch. **B** Positioning for the vertex occlusal from the front; note the use of the protective thyroid shield. **C** Positioning from the side. **D** Diagram showing the positioning from the side.

Resultant radiograph

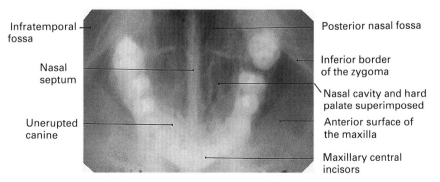

Fig. 10.6 An example of a vertex occlusal radiograph with the main radiographic features indicated.

Lower 90° occlusal

This projection shows a plan view of the tooth-bearing portion of the mandible and the floor of the mouth. A minor variation of the technique is also used to show unilateral lesions.

Main clinical indications

- Detection of the presence and position of radiopaque calculi in the submandibular salivary ducts
- Assessment of the bucco-lingual position of unerupted mandibular teeth
- Evaluation of the bucco-lingual expansion of the body of the mandible by cysts, tumours or osteodystrophies
- Assessment of displacement fractures of the anterior body of the mandible in the horizontal plane.

Fig. 10.7A Diagram showing the position of the film packet (white pebbly surface facing downwards) in relation to the lower arch. **B** Positioning for the lower 90° occlusal from the side. **C** Diagram showing the positioning from the side.

Technique and positioning

1. The film packet, with the white (pebbly) surface facing downwards, is placed centrally into the mouth, on to the occlusal surfaces of the lower teeth, with its long axis crossways. The patient is asked to bite together gently.

2. The patient *then* leans forwards and *then* tips the head backwards as far as is comfortable, where it is supported.

3. The X-ray tubehead, with circular collimator fitted, is placed below the patient's chin, in the midline, centring on an imaginary line joining the first molars, at an angle of 90° to the film (see Fig. 10.7).

Variation of technique. To show a particular part of the mandible, the film packet is placed in the mouth with its long axis anteroposteriorly over the area of interest. The X-ray tubehead, still aimed at 90° to the film, is centred below the body of the mandible in that area.

Note: The lower 90° occlusal is mounted as if the examiner were looking into the patient's mouth. The radiograph is therefore mounted with the embossed dot pointing *away* from the examiner.

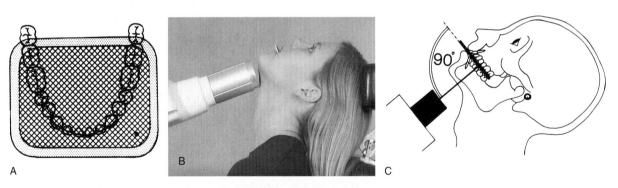

A   B   C

Resultant radiograph

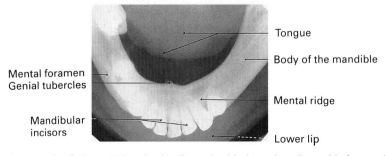

Tongue

Body of the mandible

Mental ridge

Lower lip

Mental foramen
Genial tubercles

Mandibular incisors

Fig. 10.8 An example of a lower 90° occlusal radiograph with the main radiographic features indicated.

Lower 45° occlusal

This projection is taken to show the lower anterior teeth and the anterior part of the mandible. The resultant radiograph resembles a large bisected angle technique periapical of this region.

Main clinical indications

- Periapical assessment of the lower incisor teeth, especially useful in adults and children unable to tolerate periapical films
- Evaluation of the size and extent of lesions such as cysts or tumours affecting the anterior part of the mandible
- Assessment of displacement fractures of the anterior mandible in the vertical plane.

Technique and positioning

1. The patient is seated with the head supported and with the occlusal plane horizontal and parallel to the floor.

2. The film packet, with the white (pebbly) surface facing downwards, is placed centrally into the mouth, on to the occlusal surfaces of the lower teeth, with its long axis anteroposteriorly, and the patient is asked to bite gently together.

3. The X-ray tubehead is positioned in the midline, centring through the chin point, at an angle of 45° to the film (see Fig. 10.9).

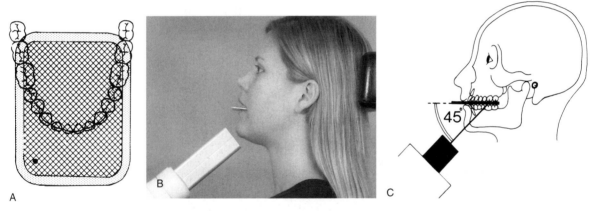

Fig. 10.9A Diagram showing the position of the film packet (white pebbly surface facing downwards) in relation to the lower arch. **B** Positioning for the lower 45° occlusal from the side. **C** Diagram showing the positioning from the side.

Resultant radiograph

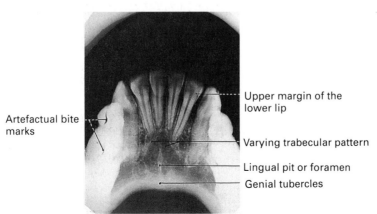

Fig. 10.10 An example of a lower 45° occlusal radiograph with the main radiographic features indicated.

Lower oblique occlusal

This projection is designed to allow the image of the submandibular salivary gland, on the side of interest, to be projected on to the film. However, because the X-ray beam is oblique, all the anatomical tissues shown are distorted.

Main indications

The main clinical indications include:

- Detection of radiopaque calculi in a submandibular salivary gland
- Assessment of the bucco-lingual position of unerupted lower wisdom teeth
- Evaluation of the extent and expansion of cysts, tumours or osteodystrophies in the posterior part of the body and angle of the mandible.

Technique and positioning

The technique can be summarized as follows:

1. The film packet, with the white (pebbly) surface facing downwards, is inserted into the mouth, on to the occlusal surfaces of the lower teeth, over to the side under investigation, with its long axis anteroposteriorly. The patient is asked to bite together gently.

2. The patient's head is supported, then rotated away from the side under investigation and the chin is raised. This rotated positioning allows the subsequent positioning of the X-ray tubehead.

3. The X-ray tubehead with circular collimator is aimed upwards and forwards towards the film, from below and behind the angle of the mandible and parallel to the lingual surface of the mandible (see Fig. 10.11).

Note: The lower oblique occlusal is also mounted with the embossed dot pointing *away* from the examiner.

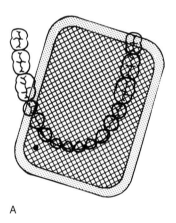

A

Resultant radiograph

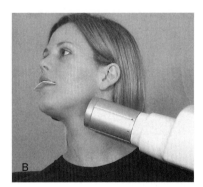

B

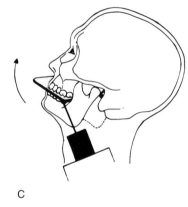

C

Fig. 10.11A Diagram showing the position of the film packet (white pebbly surface facing downwards) in relation to the lower arch for the LEFT lower oblique occlusal. **B** Positioning for the LEFT lower oblique occlusal from the side. **C** Diagram showing the positioning from the side and indicating that the patient's chin is raised and that the head is rotated AWAY from the side under investigation.

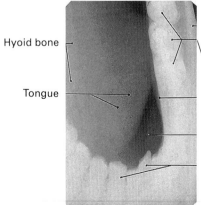

Hyoid bone

Tongue

Buccal plate of the mandible

Mandibular molars

Lingual plate of the mandible

Floor of the mouth

Mandibular incisors

Fig. 10.12 An example of a lower oblique occlusal radiograph with the main radiographic features indicated.

11 Oblique lateral radiography

Introduction

Oblique lateral radiographs are extraoral views of the jaws that can be taken using a dental X-ray set (see Fig. 11.1). Before the development of dental panoramic equipment they were the routine extraoral radiographs used both in hospitals and in general practice. In recent years, their popularity has waned, but the limitations of dental panoramic tomographs (see Ch. 13) have ensured that oblique lateral radiographs still have an important role.

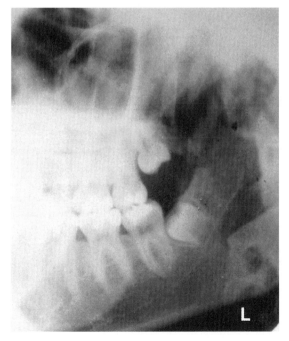

Fig. 11.1 An example of an oblique lateral showing the left molars.

Terminology

Lateral radiographs of the head and jaws are divided into:

- True laterals
- Oblique laterals
- Bimolars (two oblique laterals on one film).

The differentiating adjectives *true* and *oblique* are used to indicate the relationship of the film, patient and X-ray beam, as shown in Figure 11.2.

True lateral positioning

The film and the sagittal plane of the patient's head are parallel and the X-ray beam is perpendicular to both of them. This is the positioning for the *true lateral skull radiograph* taken in a cephalostat unit described in Chapter 12.

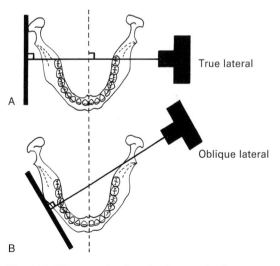

Fig. 11.2 Diagrams showing what is meant by the terms *true* and *oblique* lateral.

Oblique lateral positioning

The film and the sagittal plane of the patient's head are **not** parallel. The X-ray beam is aimed perpendicular to the film but is *oblique* to the sagittal plane of the patient. A variety of different *oblique lateral* projections is possible with different head and X-ray beam positions.

Main indications

The main clinical indications for oblique lateral radiographs include:

- Assessment of the presence and/or position of unerupted teeth
- Detection of fractures of the mandible
- Evaluation of lesions or conditions affecting the jaws including cysts, tumours, giant cell lesions, and osteodystrophies
- As an alternative when intraoral views are unobtainable because of severe gagging or if the patient is unable to open the mouth or is unconscious (see Ch. 7, Fig. 7.1)
- As specific views of the salivary glands or temporomandibular joint.

Equipment required

This includes (see Fig. 11.3):

- A dental X-ray set
- An extraoral cassette (usually 15 × 18 cm)
- A lead shield to cover half the cassette when taking bimolar views.

Specially constructed angle boards can be used to facilitate positioning, but are not considered necessary by the author.

Basic technique principles

As stated, a wide range of different oblique lateral projections of the jaws are possible. However, all the variations rely on the same basic principles regarding the position of:

- The cassette
- The patient's head
- The X-ray tubehead.

Cassette position

The cassette is held by the patient against the side of the face overlying the area of the jaws under investigation. The exact position of the cassette is determined by the area of interest.

Patient's head position

The patient is normally seated upright in the dental chair and is then instructed to:

1. *Rotate the head to the side of interest.* This is done to bring the contra-lateral ramus forwards, avoiding its superimposition and to increase the

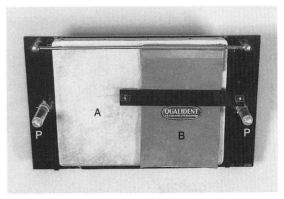

(i) (ii)

Fig. 11.3 Equipment used for oblique lateral radiography. **(i)** An 11 × 18 cm cassette **A** and lead shield **B**. **(ii)** An example of an angle board showing the cassette **A**, lead shield **B** and the plastic earpieces **P** for patient positioning.

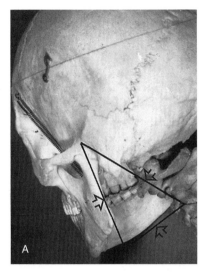 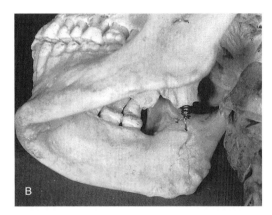

Fig. 11.4A The view through the *radiographic keyhole* (arrowed) showing the right mandibular and maxillary posterior teeth. Note the anterior teeth are obscured by the left ramus of the mandible. **B** The view from underneath the left body of the mandible showing the right mandible and right posterior mandibular teeth. Note the right maxillary teeth are obscured by the left body of the mandible.

space available between the neck and shoulder in which to position the X-ray set.

2. *Raise the chin.* This is done to increase the triangular space between the back of the ramus and the cervical spine (the so-called *radiographic keyhole*, see Fig. 11.4) through which the X-ray beam will pass.

X-ray tubehead position

The X-ray tubehead is positioned on the opposite side of the patient's head to the cassette. There are two basic positions, depending on the area of the jaws under investigation:

- *Behind the ramus aiming through the radiographic keyhole*. The X-ray tubehead is positioned along the line of the occlusal plane, just below the ear, behind the ramus aiming through the *radiographic keyhole* at the particular maxillary **and** mandibular teeth under investigation. The view from this position is illustrated in Figure 11.4A.

As shown, the X-ray beam will not pass directly between the contact areas of the posterior teeth. This may result in some overlapping of the crowns.

- *Beneath the lower border of the mandible*. The X-ray tubehead is positioned beneath the lower border of the contra-lateral body of the mandible, directly opposite the particular mandibular teeth under investigation, aiming slightly upwards. The view from this position is illustrated in Figure 11.4B. As shown, the X-ray beam will now pass between the contact areas of the teeth. However, there will still be some distortion of the image in the vertical plane owing to the upward angulation of the X-ray beam. In addition, the shadow of the body of the mandible will be superimposed over the maxillary teeth.

Once these principles are understood, the technique becomes straightforward and can be modified readily for different anatomical regions and clinical situations.

Positioning examples for various oblique lateral radiographs

Examples of the required positioning for different oblique laterals and the resultant radiographs are shown in Figures 11.5–11.8. Illustrations show the positioning for both adults and children.

Important points to note

- For stability, a small child is usually rotated through 90° in the chair, so the shoulder is supported and the cassette and head can be rested on the headrest.
- The area under investigation determines the position of the cassette and the X-ray tubehead.
- An X-ray request for an oblique lateral must specify the **exact** region of the jaws required.

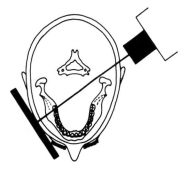

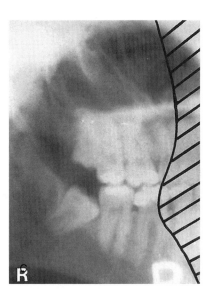

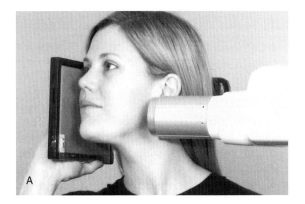

Fig. 11.5A Cassette and X-ray tubehead positions for the RIGHT mandibular **and** maxillary molars on an adult. **B** Diagram of the positioning from above showing the cassette overlying the molar teeth and the X-ray beam passing between the cervical spine and mandibular ramus. **C** A typical resultant radiograph. The shadow of the superimposed left ramus, overlying the premolars, has been drawn in to emphasize its position. Compare with Figure 11.4A. Note the radiograph is mounted and viewed as if the observer is looking at the patient from the tooth side not the other side.

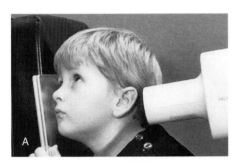

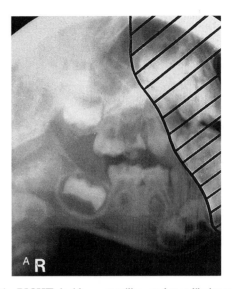

Fig. 11.6A Positioning of a child, cassette and X-ray tubehead for the RIGHT deciduous maxillary and mandibular molars. **B** A typical resultant radiograph. The shadow of the superimposed left ramus has been drawn in.

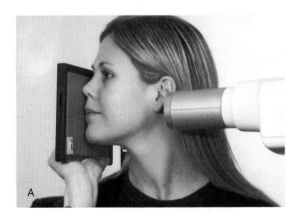

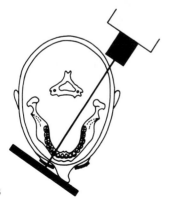

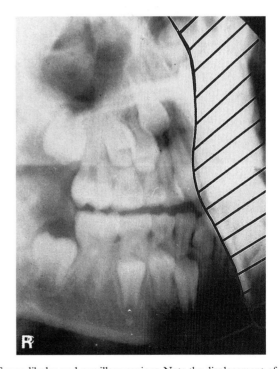

Fig. 11.7A Cassette and X-ray tubehead positions for the RIGHT mandibular and maxillary canines. Note the displacement of the nose needed to achieve the desired position for the cassette. **B** Diagram of the positioning from above, showing the cassette overlying the canine teeth and the X-ray tubehead aimed through the *radiographic keyhole*. **C** A typical resultant radiograph of a patient in the mixed dentition. The shadow of the superimposed left ramus has been drawn in—it now overlies the lateral incisors. Again note the orientation of the radiograph and how it is mounted.

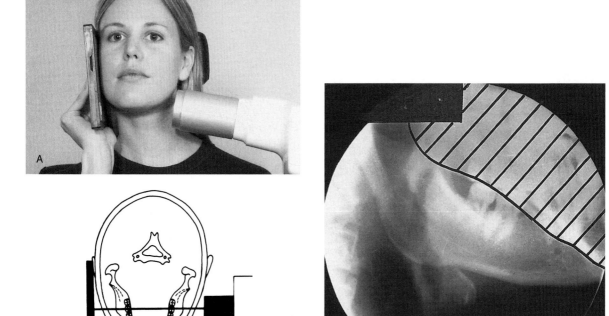

Fig. 11.8A Cassette and X-ray tubehead position for the RIGHT mandibular molars. Note the upward angulation of the X-ray tubehead and its position beneath the left body of the mandible. **B** Diagram of the positioning from above. Note the position of the X-ray tubehead and compare with Figure 11.5**B**. **C** A typical resultant radiograph showing the right mandibular molars. The superimposed shadow of the left mandibular body has been drawn in overlying the maxillary molars. Compare with Figure 11.4**B**.

Bimolar technique

As mentioned earlier, *bimolar* is the term used for the radiographic projection showing oblique lateral views of the right and left sides of the jaws on the different halves of the **same** radiograph.

The technique can be summarized as follows:

1. The patient is positioned with one side of the face in the middle of one half of the cassette, with the nose towards the midline. The precise positioning depends on which teeth or area of the jaws are being examined (like any other oblique lateral).

2. The other half of the cassette is covered by a lead shield to prevent exposure of this side of the film.

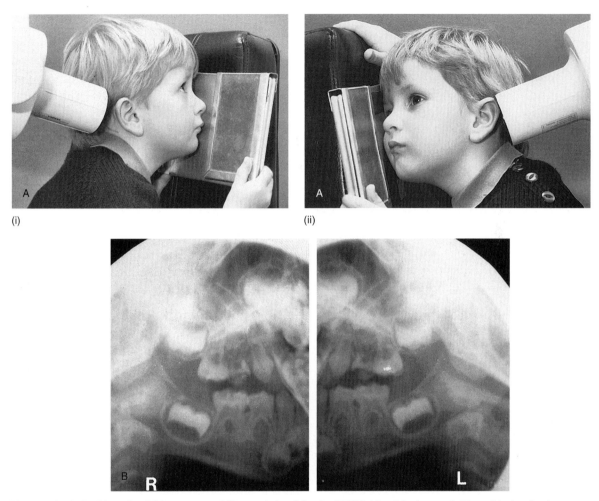

(i) (ii)

Fig. 11.9A (i) Position of a child, cassette and X-ray tubehead for the LEFT side of the jaws and **(ii)** positioning for the RIGHT side. Note the lead shield covering the half of the cassette not being used. **B** An example of a child's bimolar.

3. The X-ray tubehead is positioned to show the desired area, and the exposure is made.

4. The lead shield is then placed over the other side of the cassette to protect the part of the film already exposed.

5. The patient is then positioned in a similar manner with the cassette held on the other side of the face.

6. The X-ray tubehead is re-positioned and a second exposure made.

12 Cephalometric radiography

Cephalometric radiography is a standardized and reproducible form of skull radiography used extensively in orthodontics to assess the relationships of the teeth to the jaws and the jaws to the rest of the facial skeleton. Standardization was essential for the development of *cephalometry* — the measurement and comparison of specific points, distances and lines within the facial skeleton, which is now an integral part of orthodontic assessment. The greatest value is probably obtained from these radiographs if they are traced or digitized and this is essential when they are being used for the monitoring of treatment progress.

Main indications

The main clinical indications can be considered under two major headings — orthodontics and orthognathic surgery.

Orthodontics

- Initial diagnosis — confirmation of the underlying skeletal and/or soft tissue abnormalities
- Treatment planning
- Monitoring treatment progress, e.g. to assess anchorage requirements and incisor inclination
- Appraisal of treatment results, e.g. 1 or 2 months before the completion of active treatment to ensure that treatment targets have been met and to allow planning of retention.

When considering these indications, it should be remembered that all radiographs must be clinically justified under current legislation (see Ch. 6). Indications and selection criteria for cephalometric radiographs are clearly identified in the Faculty of General Dental Practitioners *Selection Criteria in Dental Radiography* booklet published in the UK in 1998 and in the British Orthodontic Society's booklet *Guidelines for the Use of Radiographs in Clinical Orthodontics*, published in the UK in 2001. These guidelines are designed to assist in the *justification* process so as to avoid the use of unnecessary radiographs.

Orthognathic surgery

- Preoperative evaluation of skeletal and soft tissue patterns
- To assist in treatment planning
- Postoperative appraisal of the results of surgery and long-term follow-up studies.

Equipment

Several different types of equipment are available for cephalometric radiography, either as separate units, or as additional attachments to dental panoramic units. In some equipment, the patients are seated, while in others they remain standing. Despite these variables the essential requirements for this type of equipment are the same and include:

- *Cephalostat* (or *craniostat*) (see Fig. 12.1) comprising:
  — Head positioning and stabilizing apparatus with ear rods to ensure a standardized patient position (some units also have infra-orbital guide rods)

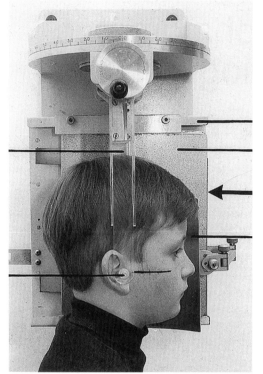

Cassette holder

Fixed anti-scatter grid

Cassette positioned behind the grid

Aluminium wedge

Head stabilizing and positioning apparatus

Ear rod

Fig. 12.1 A typical cephalostat (craniostat) containing a patient with the main features indicated. Note that this design of cephalostat has the aluminium wedge filter positioned between the patient and the anti-scatter grid. The Frankfort plane is marked on the patient's face.

— Fixed anti-scatter grid — to stop photons scattered within the patient reaching the film and degrading the final image
— Cassette holder.
- *Cassette* (usually 18 × 24 cm) containing intensifying screens and indirect-action film.
- *Aluminium wedge filter.* This is either part of the cephalostat and positioned between the patient and the anterior part of the cassette, as shown in Figure 12.1, or it is attached to the tubehead, covering the anterior part of the emerging beam. Its function is to attenuate the X-ray beam selectively in the region of the facial soft tissues because these tissues are not dense enough on their own to produce a visible radiographic shadow. This added attenuation enables the soft tissue profile to be seen on the final radiograph.

- *X-ray generating apparatus* that should be:
— In a fixed position relative to the cephalostat (approx. 2 m) and the film (see Fig. 12.2) so that successive radiographs are reproducible and comparable
— Capable of producing an X-ray beam that is:
  * Sufficiently penetrating to reach the film
  * Parallel in nature to minimize magnification between R and L sides of the mandible and to ensure that the midline points S, N and A are as sharp as possible
  * Collimated to an approximately triangular shape to restrict the area of the patient irradiated to the required cranial base and facial skeleton, so avoiding the skull vault and cervical spine (see Figs 12.2 and 12.3).

Main radiographic projections

These include:

- True cephalometric lateral skull
- Cephalometric postero-anterior of the jaws (PA jaws).

True cephalometric lateral skull

As stated in Chapter 11, the terminology used to describe lateral skull projections is somewhat confusing, the adjective *true*, as opposed to *oblique*, being used to describe lateral skull projections when:

- The film is parallel to the sagittal plane of the patient's head
- The X-ray beam is perpendicular to film and sagittal plane.

In addition, the word *cephalometric* should be included when describing the *true lateral skull* radiograph taken in the cephalostat. This enables differentiation from the non-standardized true lateral skull projection taken in a skull unit. It is now an accepted convention to view orthodontic lateral skull radiographs with the patient facing to the *right*, as shown in Figure 12.3.

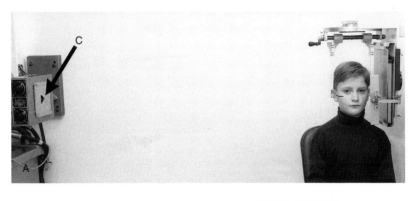

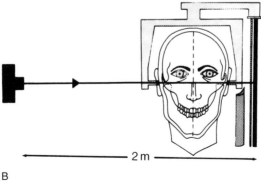

Fig. 12.2A Positioning for the true cephalometric lateral skull projection. Note the X-ray tubehead and cephalostat are in fixed positions (approximately 2 m apart) and the patient's head is stabilized within the cephalostat with the Frankfort plane horizontal. The triangular collimator (C) is indicated by the arrow. **B** Diagram of the positioning from the front — the sagittal plane of the head is parallel to the film, and the X-ray beam is horizontal and perpendicular to the sagittal plane and the film.

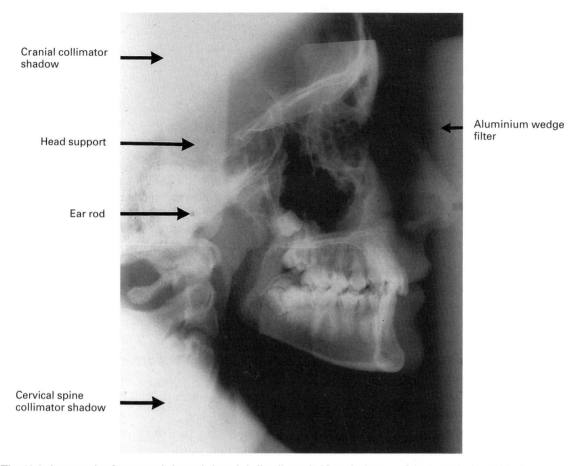

Cranial collimator shadow

Head support

Ear rod

Cervical spine collimator shadow

Aluminium wedge filter

Fig. 12.3 An example of a true cephalometric lateral skull radiograph. Note the images of the ear rods should ideally appear superimposed on one another. The various shadows of the cephalostat equipment and the collimator are indicated.

Technique and positioning

This can be summarized as follows:

1. The patient is positioned within the cephalostat, with the sagittal plane of the head vertical and parallel to the film and with the Frankfort plane horizontal. The teeth should generally be in maximum intercuspation.

2. The head is immobilized carefully within the apparatus with the plastic ear rods being inserted gradually into the external auditory meati.

3. The aluminium wedge is positioned to cover the anterior part of the film.

4. The equipment is designed to ensure that when the patient is positioned correctly, the X-ray beam is horizontal and centred on the ear rods (see Fig. 12.2).

Cephalometric tracing / digitizing

This produces a diagrammatic representation of certain anatomical points or landmarks evident on the lateral skull radiograph (see Fig. 12.4). These points are traced on to an overlying sheet of paper or acetate or digitally recorded. Either method allows precise measurements to be made. As a basic system these could include:

- The outline and inclination of the anterior teeth
- The positional relationship of the mandibular and maxillary dental bases to the cranial base
- The positional relationship of the dental bases to one another, i.e. the skeletal patterns
- The relationship between the bones of the skull and the soft tissues of the face.

Main cephalometric points

The definitions of the main cephalometric points (as indicated in a clockwise direction on the tracing shown in Fig. 12.4) include:

Sella (S). The centre of the sella turcica, (determined by inspection).

Orbitale (Or). The lowest point on the infra-orbital margin.

Nasion (N). The most anterior point on the frontonasal suture.

Anterior nasal spine (ANS). The tip of the anterior nasal spine.

Subspinale or point A. The deepest midline point between the anterior nasal spine and prosthion.

Prosthion (Pr). The most anterior point of the alveolar crest in the premaxilla, usually between the upper central incisors.

Infradentale (Id). The most anterior point of the alveolar crest, situated between the lower central incisors.

Supramentale or point B. The deepest point in the bony outline between the infradentale and the pogonion.

Pogonion (Pog). The most anterior point of the bony chin.

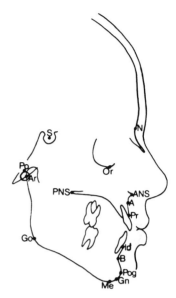

Fig. 12.4 A cephalometric tracing of a lateral skull radiograph showing the main cephalometric points.

Gnathion (Gn). The most anterior and inferior point on the bony outline of the chin, situated equidistant from pogonion and menton.

Menton (Me). The lowest point on the bony outline of the mandibular symphysis.

Gonion (Go). The most lateral external point at the junction of the horizontal and ascending rami of the mandible.

Note: The gonion is found by bisecting the angle formed by tangents to the posterior and inferior borders of the mandible.

Posterior nasal spine (PNS). The tip of the posterior spine of the palatine bone in the hard palate.

Articulare (Ar). The point of intersection of the dorsal contours of the posterior border of the mandible and temporal bone.

Porion (Po). The uppermost point of the bony external auditory meatus, usually regarded as coincidental with the uppermost point of the ear rods of the cephalostat.

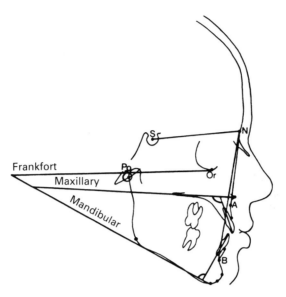

Fig. 12.5 A cephalometric tracing of a lateral skull radiograph showing the main cephalometric planes and angles.

Main cephalometric planes and angles

The definitions of the main cephalometric planes and angles shown in Figure 12.5 include:

Frankfort plane. A transverse plane through the skull represented by the line joining porion and orbitale.

Mandibular plane. A transverse plane through the skull representing the lower border of the horizontal ramus of the mandible.

There are several definitions:

- A tangent to the lower border of the mandible
- A line joining gnathion and gonion
- A line joining menton and gonion.

Maxillary plane. A transverse plane through the skull represented by a joining of the anterior and posterior nasal spines.

SN plane. A transverse plane through the skull represented by the line joining sella and nasion.

SNA. Relates the anteroposterior position of the maxilla, as represented by the A point, to the cranial base.

SNB. Relates the anteroposterior position of the mandible, as represented by the B point, to the cranial base.

ANB. Relates the anteroposterior position of the maxilla to the mandible, i.e. indicates the anteroposterior skeletal pattern — Class I, II or III.

Maxillary incisal inclination. The angle between the long axis of the maxillary incisors and the maxillary plane.

Mandibular incisal inclination. The angle between the long axis of the mandibular incisors and the mandibular plane.

All the definitions are those specified in The British Standards Glossary of Dental terms (BS4492: 1983).

Cephalometric postero-anterior of the jaws (PA jaws)

This postero-anterior (PA) view of the jaws, like the Lateral view, is standardized and reproducible. This makes it suitable for the assessment of facial asymmetries and for preoperative and postoperative comparisons in orthognathic surgery involving the mandible.

Technique and positioning

This can be summarized as follows:

1. The head-stabilizing apparatus of the cephalostat is rotated through 90°.

2. The patient is positioned in the apparatus with the head tipped forwards and with the radiographic baseline horizontal and perpendicular to the film, i.e. in the *forehead–nose* position.

3. The head is immobilized within the apparatus by inserting the plastic ear rods into the external auditory meati.

4. The fixed X-ray beam is horizontal with the central ray centred through the cervical spine at the level of the rami of the mandible (see Fig. 12.6).

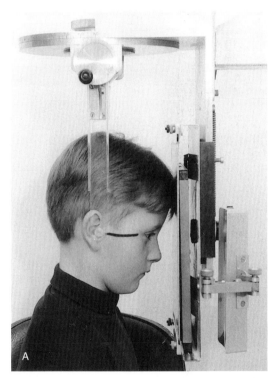

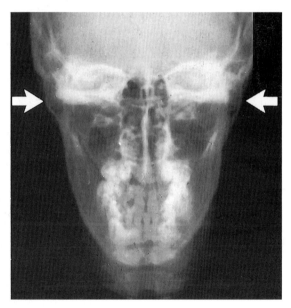

Fig. 12.7 An example of a cephalometric PA jaws radiograph. The arrows indicate the position of the ear rods.

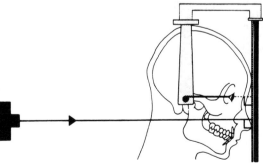

Fig. 12.6A Positioning for the cephalometric PA jaws projection. The patient is in the *forehead–nose* position, with the radiographic baseline (marked on the face) horizontal and perpendicular to the film. **B** Diagram of the patient positioning and showing the X-ray beam horizontal and centred through the rami.

13 Dental panoramic tomography

Introduction

Dental panoramic tomography has become a very popular radiographic technique in dentistry. The main reasons for this include:

- All the teeth and their supporting structures are shown on one film (see Fig. 13.1)

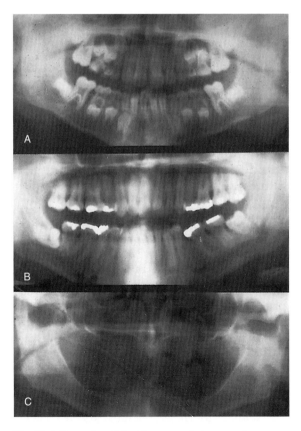

Fig. 13.1 Examples of dental panoramic tomographs (DPTs). **A** A child in mixed dentition. **B** A dentate adult. **C** An edentulous adult.

- The technique is reasonably simple
- The radiation dose is relatively low, particularly with modern DC units with rare-earth intensifying screens — the dose is equivalent to about three to four perapical radiographs.

The major drawback to the technique is that the resultant film is a *sectional radiograph*, and like all other forms of *tomography* only structures within the *section* will be evident and in focus on the final film. In panoramic tomography, the *section* or *focal trough* is designed to be approximately horseshoe shaped, corresponding to the shape of the dental arches. Unfortunately, the image quality is inferior to that of intraoral (periapical and bitewing) radiographs and interpretation is more complicated, as described later.

Selection criteria

In the UK, the *Selection Criteria in Dental Radiography* booklet recommends a dental panoramic tomograph (DPT) in general dental practice in the following circumstances:

- As part of an orthodontic assessment where there is a clinical need to know the state of the dentition and the presence/absence of teeth
- To assess bony lesions or an unerupted tooth that are too large to be demonstrated on intraoral films
- Prior to dental surgery under general anaesthesia
- As part of an assessment of periodontal bone support where there is pocketing greater than 5 mm
- Assessment of third molars, at a time when consideration needs to be given to whether they should be removed or not.

In addition, in dental hospitals DPTs are also used to assess:

- Fractures of all parts of the mandible except the anterior region
- Antral disease — particularly to the floor, posterior and medial walls of the antra
- Destructive diseases of the articular surfaces of the TMJ
- Vertical alveolar bone height as part of pre-implant planning.

The *Selection Criteria* booklet specifically states that 'panoramic radiographs should only be taken in the presence of clinical signs and symptoms', and goes on to say that 'there is no justification for review panoramic examinations at arbitrary intervals' (see Ch. 6 on *justification*).

Theory

The theory of dental panoramic tomography is complicated. Nevertheless, an understanding of how the resultant radiographic image is produced and which structures are in fact being imaged is necessary for a critical evaluation and for the interpretation of this type of radiograph.

The difficulty in panoramic tomography arises from the need to produce a final shape of focal trough which approximates to the shape of the dental arches.

An explanation of how this final horseshoe-shaped focal trough is achieved is given below. But first, other types of tomography — which form the basis of panoramic tomography — are described, showing how they result in different shapes of focal trough. These include:

- Linear tomography using a wide or broad X-ray beam
- Linear tomography using a narrow or slit X-ray beam
- Rotational tomography using a slit X-ray beam.

Broad-beam linear tomography

This is illustrated in Figure 13.2. The synchronized movement of the tubehead and film, in the *vertical* plane, results in a straight linear focal trough. The broad X-ray beam exposes the entire film throughout the exposure.

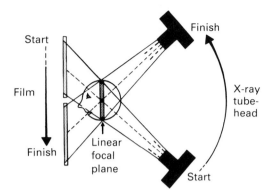

Fig. 13.2 Diagram showing the theory of broad-beam linear tomography to produce a vertical coronal section with the synchronized movement of the X-ray tubehead and the film in the vertical plane. Using a broad beam, there will be multiple centres of rotation (three are indicated: •), all of which will lie in the shaded zone. As all these centres of rotation will be in focus, this zone represents the focal plane or section that will appear in focus on the resultant tomograph. **Note** — the broad X-ray beam exposes the **entire** film throughout the exposure.

Slit or narrow-beam linear tomography

A similar straight linear tomograph can also be produced by modifying the equipment and using a narrow or slit X-ray beam. The equipment is designed so that the narrow beam traverses the film exposing different parts of the film during the tomographic movement. Only by the end of the tomographic movement has the entire film been exposed. The following equipment modifications are necessary:

- The X-ray beam has to be collimated from a broad beam to a narrow beam.
- The film cassette has to be placed behind a protective metal shield. A narrow opening in this shield is required to allow a small part of the film to be exposed to the X-ray beam at any one instant.
- A cassette carrier, incorporating the metal shield, has to be linked to the X-ray tubehead to ensure that they move in the **opposite** direction to one another during the exposure. This produces the synchronized tomographic movement in the *vertical* plane.
- Within this carrier, the film cassette itself has to be moved in the **same** direction as the tubehead. This ensures that a different part of the film is exposed to the X-ray beam throughout the exposure.

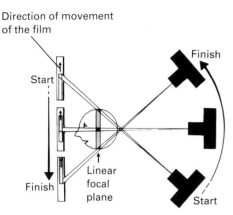

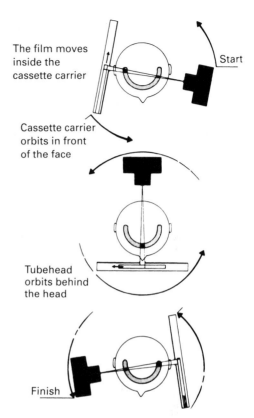

Fig. 13.3 Diagram showing the theory of narrow-beam linear tomography to produce a vertical coronal section. The tomographic movement is produced by the synchronized movement of the X-ray tubehead and the cassette carrier, in the vertical plane. The film, placed behind the metal protective front of the cassette carrier, also moves during the exposure, in the same direction as the X-ray tubehead. The narrow X-ray beam traverses the patient and film, exposing a **different** part of the film throughout the cycle.

The principle of narrow-beam linear tomography using this equipment is illustrated in Figure 13.3.

Narrow beam rotational tomography

In this type of tomography, narrow-beam equipment is again used, but the synchronized movement of the X-ray tubehead and the cassette carrier are designed to rotate in the *horizontal* plane, in a *circular* path around the head, with a *single* centre of rotation. The resultant focal trough is curved and forms the arc of a circle, as shown in Figure 13.4.

Important points to note

- The X-ray tubehead orbits around the **back** of the head while the cassette carrier with the film orbits around the **front** of the face.
- The X-ray tubehead and the cassette carrier move in **opposite** directions to one another.
- The film moves in the **same** direction as the X-ray tubehead, behind the protective metal shield of the cassette carrier.
- A different part of the film is exposed to the X-ray beam at any one instant, as the equipment orbits the head.

Fig. 13.4 Diagrams showing the theory of narrow beam rotational tomography. The tomographic movement is provided by the circular synchronized movement of the X-ray tubehead in one direction and the cassette carrier in the opposite direction, in the horizontal plane. The equipment has a single centre of rotation. The film also moves inside the cassette carrier so that a **different** part of the film is exposed to the narrow beam during the cycle, thus by the end the entire film has been exposed. The focal plane or trough (shaded) is curved and forms the arc of a circle.

- The simple circular rotational movement with a single centre of rotation produces a curved **circular** focal trough.
- As in conventional tomography, shadows of structures not within the focal trough will be out of focus and blurred owing to the tomographic movement.

Dental panoramic tomography

The dental arch, though curved, is not the shape of an arc of a circle. To produce the required elliptical, horseshoe-shaped focal trough, panoramic tomographic equipment employs the principle of narrow-beam rotational tomography, but uses two or more centres of rotation.

There are several dental panoramic units available; they all work on the same principle but differ in how the rotational movement is modified to image the elliptical dental arch. Four main methods (see Fig. 13.5) have been used including:

- Two stationary centres of rotation, using two separate circular arcs
- Three stationary centres of rotation, using three separate circular arcs
- A continually moving centre of rotation using multiple circular arcs combined to form a final elliptical shape
- A combination of three stationary centres of rotation and a moving centre of rotation.

However the focal troughs are produced, it should be remembered that they are three-dimensional. The focal trough is thus sometimes described as a *focal corridor*. All structures within the corridor, including the mandibular and maxillary teeth, will be in focus on the final radiograph. The vertical height of the corridor is determined by the shape and height of the X-ray beam and the size of the film as shown in Figure 13.6.

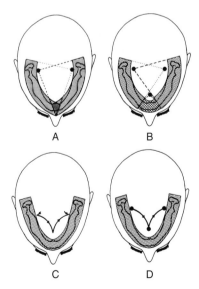

Fig. 13.5 Diagrams showing the main methods that have been used to produce a focal trough that approximates to the elliptical shape of the dental arch using different centres of rotation. **A** 2 stationary, **B** 3 stationary, **C** continually moving, **D** combination of 3 stationary and moving centre.

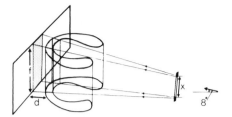

Fig. 13.6 Diagram showing how the height of the three-dimensional focal corridor is determined. The height (x) of the X-ray beam is collimated to just cover the height (f) of the film. The separation of the focal trough and the film (d), coupled with the 8° upward angulation of the X-ray beam results in the final image being slightly magnified.

As in other forms of narrow-beam tomography, a different part of the focal trough is imaged throughout the exposure. The final radiograph is thus built up of sections (see Fig. 13.7), each created separately, as the equipment orbits around the patient's head.

Equipment

There are several different dental panoramic tomographic units available. Although varying in design, all consist of three main components, namely:

- An *X-ray tubehead*, producing a narrow fan-shaped X-ray beam, angled upwards at approximately 8° to the horizontal (see Fig. 13.6)
- A *cassette* and *cassette carriage assembly*
- *Patient-positioning apparatus* including light beam markers.

Examples of two typical machines are shown in Figure 13.8. Regulations relating to panoramic equipment are summarised in Chapter 6.

Almost all modern panoramic machines have a continuous-mode of operation and produce a so-called *continuous* image showing an uninterrupted image of the jaws, as described below. However, one machine was developed that produced a so-called *split-mode* image because the radiographic image is split by a broad, vertical, white, unexposed zone, with duplication of the midline, as shown in Figure 13.9. The split-mode equipment is now only of historical interest, but split-mode images may still be encountered in patients' records.

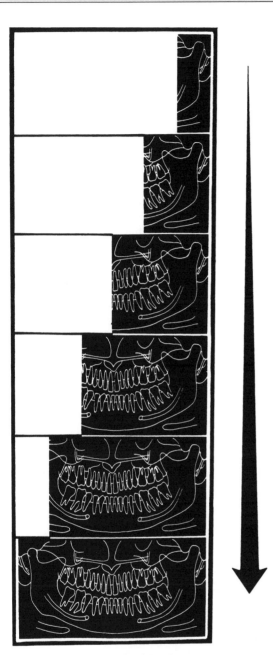

Fig. 13.7 Diagram showing the gradual build-up of a panoramic tomograph over an 18-second cycle, illustrating how a different part of the patient is imaged at different stages in the cycle.

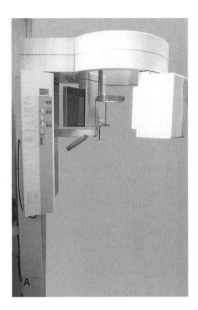

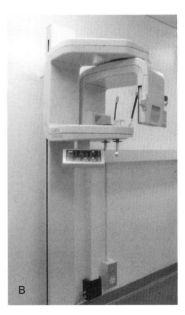

Fig. 13.8 Examples of two dental panoramic tomography machines. The basic components common to both machines include the X-ray tubehead, cassette carrier and the patient positioning apparatus.

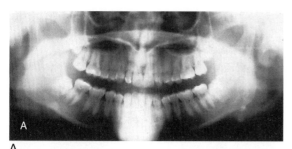

A

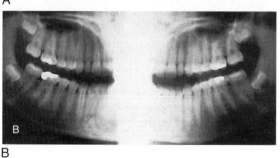

B

Fig. 13.9A A *continuous-mode* dental panoramic tomograph. **B** A *split-mode* dental panoramic tomograph, showing each side of the jaws shown separately on either side of the film and with duplication of structures near the midline.

Continuous-mode equipment

X-ray production is continuous throughout an uninterrupted tomographic cycle, during which the centres of rotation are adjusted automatically. A diagrammatic example of how a typical machine functions is shown in Figure 13.10.

Technique and positioning

The exact positioning techniques vary from one machine to another. However, there are some general requirements that are common to all machines and these can be summarized as follows:

- Patients should be asked to remove any earrings, jewellery, hair pins, spectacles, dentures or orthodontic appliances.
- The procedure and equipment movements should be explained, to reassure patients.

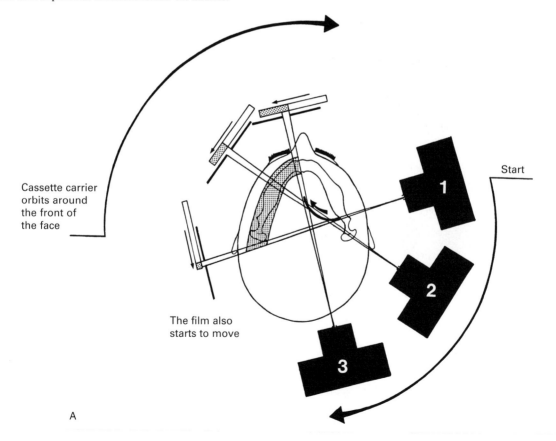

A

- A protective lead apron should **not** be used. The NRPB/RCR *Guidelines on Radiology Standards in Primary Dental Care* (1994) positively discourage the use of lead aprons because they can interfere with the final image (see Ch. 6 and Fig. 13.23F).
- Patients should be placed accurately within the machines using the various head-positioning devices and light-beam marker positioning guides (see Fig. 13.11). (In some units the patients face away from the equipment and towards the operator and in others the patient faces the other way round.)
- Patients should be instructed to place their tongue into the roof of the mouth so that it is in contact with the hard palate and **not to**

move throughout the exposure cycle (approximately 18 seconds).
- Appropriate exposure setting should be selected, typically in the range 70–100 kV and 4–12 mA.

Note: Panoramic tomography is generally considered to be unsuitable for children under 5 years old, because of the length of the exposure and the need for the patient to keep still.

The importance of accurate patient positioning

The positioning of the patient's head within this type of equipment is critical — it must be

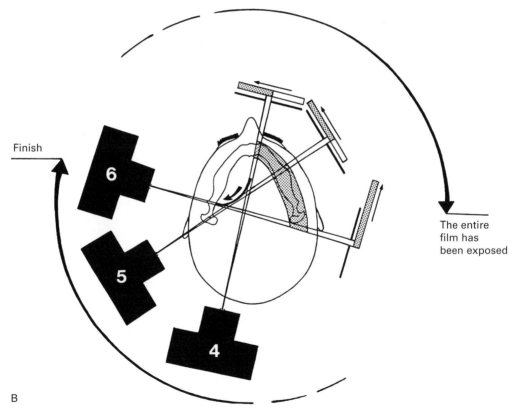

Fig. 13.10 Diagrams from above, showing the relative movements of the X-ray tubehead, cassette carrier and film during an exposure cycle of a continuous-mode panoramic unit. **A** Initially the left side of the jaw is imaged (position 1). As the X-ray tubehead moves behind the patient's head to image the anterior teeth, the cassette carrier moves in front of the patient's face and the centre of rotation moves forward along the dark arc (arrowed) towards the midline. **B** The X-ray tubehead and cassette carrier continue to move around the patient's head to image the opposite side and the centre of rotation moves backwards along the dark arc (arrowed) away from the midline. Throughout the cycle, the film is also continuously moving as illustrated, so that a different part of the film is being exposed at any one moment.

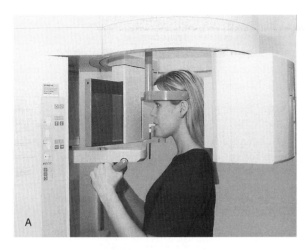

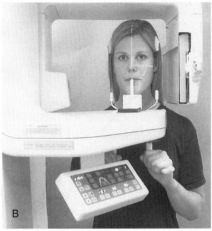

Fig. 13.11A Patient positioned in the Siemens Orthophos. **B** Patient positioned in the Planmeca PM2002. Note the bite-peg, chin and forehead or temporal supports to facilitate positioning. Slight-beam marker lines are also provided as shown in **B**.

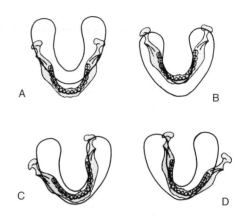

Fig. 13.12 Diagrams showing the position of the mandible in relation to the focal trough when the patient is not positioned correctly. **A** The patient is too close to the film and in front of the focal trough. **B** The patient is too far away from the film and behind the focal trough. **C** and **D** The patient is placed asymmetrically within the machine.

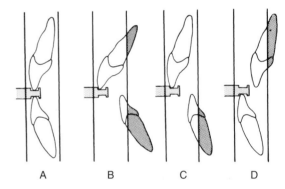

Fig. 13.13 Diagrams showing the vertical walls of the focal trough in the incisor region and the relative positions of the teeth with different underlying dental or skeletal abnormalities. **A** Class I. **B** Gross class II division 1 malocclusion with large overjet. **C** Angle's class II skeletal base. **D** Angle's class III skeletal base. The shaded areas outside the focal trough will be blurred and out of focus.

positioned accurately so that the teeth lie within the *focal trough*. The effects of placing the head too far forward, too far back or asymmetrically in relation to the focal trough, are shown in Figure 13.12. The parts of the jaws outside the focal trough will be out of focus. The fan-shaped X-ray beam causes patient malposition to be represented mainly as distortion in the horizontal plane, i.e. teeth appear too wide or too narrow rather than foreshortened or elongated. These and other positioning errors are shown later (see Fig. 13.24).

However accurately the patient's head is positioned, the inclination of the incisor teeth, or the underlying skeletal base pattern, may make it impossible to position both the mandibular **and** maxillary teeth ideally within the focal corridor (see Fig. 13.13).

Field limitation techniques

A recent development in panoramic tomography is the ability to programme the equipment to only X-ray certain parts of the jaws when specific

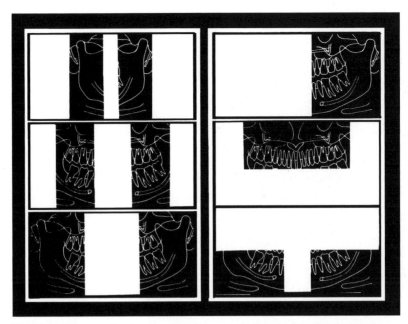

Fig. 13.14 Diagram showing a variety of segmental panoramic images that can be obtained using the newly developed field limitation techniques. As illustrated, only preselected parts of the patient are exposed and imaged on the final panoramic film.

information is required, instead of the entire dentition. This results in a significant radiation dose reduction. A variety of these so-called *field limitation techniques* are possible and a selection is illustrated in Figure 13.14.

Normal anatomy

The normal anatomical shadows that are evident on panoramic radiographs vary from one machine to another, but in general they can be subdivided into:

- *Real* or *actual shadows* of structures in, or close to, the focal trough
- *Ghost* or *artefactual shadows* created by the tomographic movement and cast by structures on the opposite side or a long way from the focal trough. The 8° upward angulation of the X-ray beam means that these ghost shadows appear at a higher level than the structures that have caused them.

These two types of shadows are clearly demonstrated in Figures 13.15 and 13.16.

Real or actual shadows

Important hard tissue shadows
(see Fig. 13.17)

These include:

- Teeth
- Mandible
- Maxilla, including the floor, medial and posterior walls of the antra
- Hard palate
- Zygomatic arches
- Styloid processes
- Hyoid bone
- Nasal septum and conchae
- Orbital rim
- Base of skull.

An additional real shadow is often cast by the vertical plastic head supports.

Air shadows

- Mouth/oral opening
- Oropharynx.

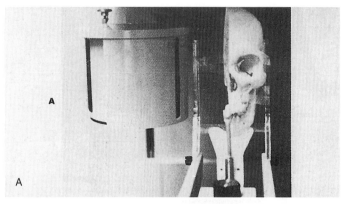

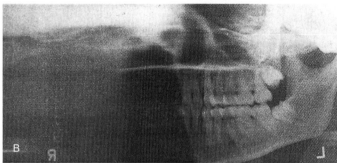

Fig. 13.15A Hemisectioned skull positioned in a dental panoramic machine. **B** Resultant radiograph showing the **real** shadows on the left and the radiopaque **ghost** shadows on the right. (Reproduced from *Oral Radiology*, by kind permission of Paul W. Goaz and Stuart C. White and The C. V. Mosby Company.)

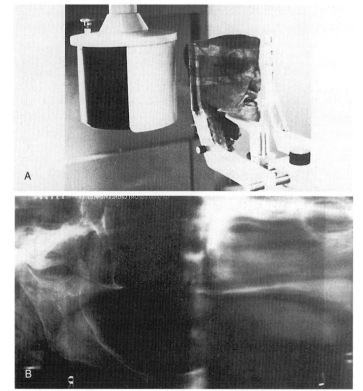

Fig. 13.16A Hemisected cadaver head positioned in a dental panoramic machine. **B** Resultant radiograph showing the real hard and soft tissue shadows on the right and the ghost shadows on the left. (Reproduced from *Oral Radiology*, by kind permission of Paul W. Goaz and Stuart C. White and The C.V. Mosby Company.)

Important soft tissue shadows (see Fig. 13.18)

- Ear lobes
- Nasal cartilages
- Soft palate
- Dorsum of tongue
- Lips and cheeks
- Nasolabial folds.

Ghost or artefactual shadows (see Fig. 13.19)

The more important ghost shadows include:

- Cervical vertebrae
- Body, angle and ramus of the contralateral side of the mandible
- Palate.

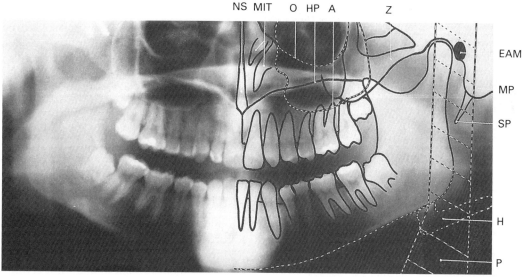

Fig. 13.17 A dental panoramic tomograph showing the main **real hard tissue** shadows, including the plastic head support, drawn in on one side of the radiograph, **NS** — nasal septum, **MIT** — middle and inferior turbinates, **O** — orbital margin, **HP** — hard palate, **A** — floor of antrum, **Z** — zygomatic arch, **EAM** — external auditory meatus, **MP** — mastoid process, **SP** — styloid process, **H** — hyoid, **P** — plastic head support.

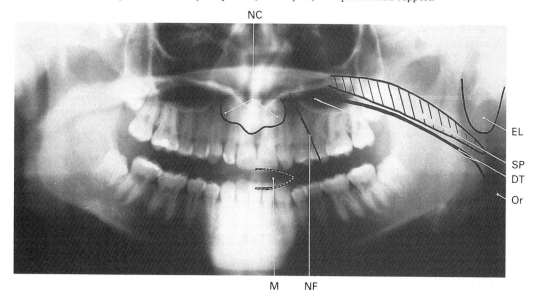

Fig. 13.18 A dental panoramic tomograph showing the main **real soft tissue** and **air** shadows drawn in on one side of the radiograph, **NC** — nasal cartilages, **EL** — ear lobe, **SP** — soft palate, **DT** — dorsum of tongue, **Or** — oropharynx, **NF** — naso-labial fold, **M** — mouth.

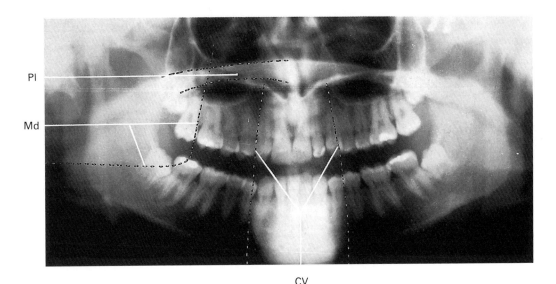

Fig. 13.19 A dental panoramic tomograph showing the main anatomical **ghost** or **artefactual shadows** drawn in on one side of the radiograph, **Pl** — palate, **Md** — mandible, **CV** — cervical vertebrae.

Advantages and disadvantages

Advantages

- A large area is imaged and all the tissues within the focal trough are displayed on one film, including the anterior teeth, even when the patient is unable to open the mouth.
- The image is easy for patients to understand, and is therefore a useful teaching aid.
- Patient movement in the vertical plane distorts only that part of the image being produced at that instant.
- Positioning is relatively simple and minimal expertise is required.
- The overall view of the jaws allows rapid assessment of any underlying, possibly unsuspected, disease.
- The view of both sides of the mandible on one film is useful when assessing fractures and is comfortable for the injured patient.
- The overall view is useful for evaluation of periodontal status and in orthodontic assessments.
- The antral floor, medial and posterior walls are well shown.
- Both condylar heads are shown on one film, allowing easy comparison.

- The radiation dose (*effective dose*) is about one-third of the dose from a full-mouth survey of intraoral films (see Ch. 3).
- Development of field limitation techniques with resultant dose reduction.

Disadvantages

- The tomographic image represents only a section of the patient. Structures or abnormalities not in the focal trough may not be evident (Fig. 13.20).
- Soft tissue and air shadows can overlie the required hard tissue structures (Fig. 13.21).
- Ghost or artefactual shadows can overlie the structures in the focal trough (Fig. 13.22).
- The tomographic movement together with the distance between the focal trough and film produce distortion and magnification of the final image (approx. × 1.3).
- The use of indirect-action film and intensifying screens results in some loss of image quality.
- The technique is not suitable for children under 5 years or on some disabled patients because of the length of the exposure cycle.
- Some patients do not conform to the shape of the focal trough and some structures will be out of focus.

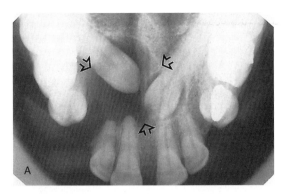

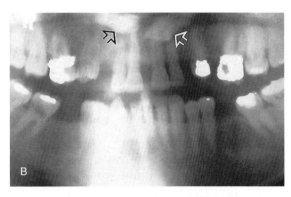

Fig. 13.20A Upper standard occlusal showing unerupted <u>3/3</u> and a large dentigerous cyst (arrowed) associated with <u>3 /</u>. **B** Dental panoramic tomograph showing the two unerupted canines out of focus (arrowed) and only a suggestion of the dentigerous cyst, because they are all outside the focal trough.

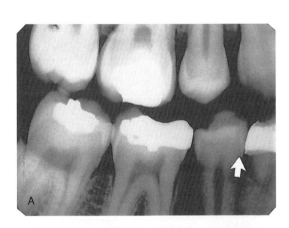

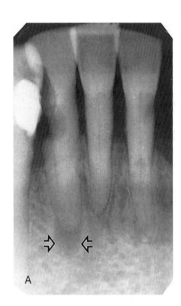

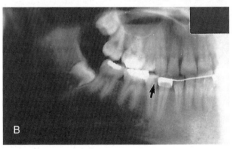

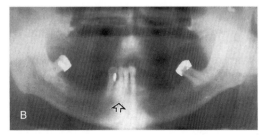

Fig. 13.21A Right bitewing showing no evidence of mesial caries in <u>5/</u> (arrowed). **B** Dental panoramic tomograph showing an apparent lesion in this tooth (arrowed). This appearance is created by the overlying air shadow of the corner of the mouth.

Fig. 13.22A Periapical of 21/12 region showing an area of radiolucency at the apex of 1/ (arrowed). **B** Dental panoramic tomograph showing no evidence of the lesion (arrowed) owing to superimposition of the shadow of the cervical vertebrae.

Errors

Examples of a variety of errors are shown in Figures 13.23–13.25 and the more common positioning errors are summarized in Table 13.1.

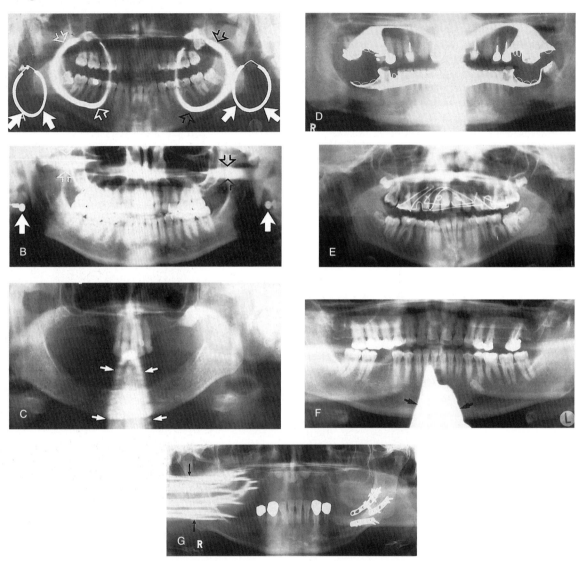

Fig. 13.23 Examples of common artefacts caused by jewellery or other objects.
A Failure to remove large ring-shaped earrings — note each earring casts two shadows, one real (in focus, solid arrows) and one ghost (blurred, open arrows). The ghost shadow of the LEFT earring is marked with open white arrows, that of the RIGHT earring with open black arrows.
B Failure to remove stud earrings, real shadows (solid arrows) with ghost shadows (open arrows).
C Failure to remove a necklace — blurred ghost shadow (arrowed).
D Failure to remove upper and lower metallic partial dentures.
E Failure to remove an upper orthodontic appliance.
F Protective lead apron placed too high on the neck, casting a dense radiopaque shadow over the anterior part of the mandible (arrowed). It is for this reason that lead aprons are positively discouraged during panoramic radiography.
G Metallic bone plates used for fixation of a fracture of the left side of the mandible casting their ghost shadows (arrowed) onto the right side of the film.

Table 13.1 Summary of common positioning errors in dental panoramic tomography and the resulting fault(s) on the film

Positioning error	Film fault
Patient too far from the film	Anterior teeth magnified in width and out of focus
Patient too close to the film	Anterior teeth narrowed and out of focus
Patient positioned asymmetrically (head turned to the right or left)	Posterior teeth enlarged on one side and reduced on the other
Patient's chin positioned too high or too low	Distortion in the shape of the mandible and the anterior teeth out of focus
Patient still wearing earrings, jewellery, dentures or orthodontic appliances	Artefactual shadow(s) of the offending object
Failure to instruct the patient to keep still throughout the cycle	Vertical or horizontal distortion of the part of the image being produced at the time of the movement

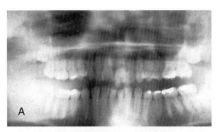

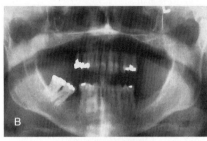

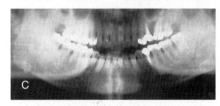

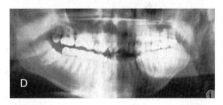

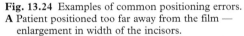

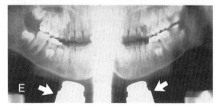

Fig. 13.24 Examples of common positioning errors.
A Patient positioned too far away from the film — enlargement in width of the incisors.
B Patient positioned too close to the film — reduction in width of the incisors. Tongue not in contact with the palate — radiolucent band across the film.
C Patient positioned with the Frankfort plane and chin tipped downwards — foreshortening of the lower incisors and increased shadowing over the posterior parts of the mandible.
D Patient placed asymmetrically in the machine — enlargement of the teeth and jaws on the right side, reduction in size on the left.
E The X-ray tubehead and film assembly positioned too low relative to the patient — the antra and condyles are not imaged but shadows of the chin rest are evident (arrowed).

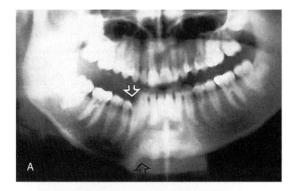

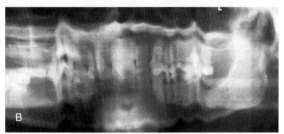

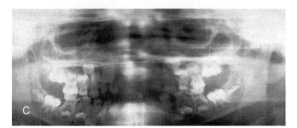

Footnote

Dental panoramic tomographs should not be considered an alternative to intraoral radiographs. However, they may be considered as an alternative to right and left *oblique lateral* radiographs or the bimolar projection (see Ch. 11) mainly because less operator expertise is required to produce adequate panoramic films.

The diagnostic value of these films is increased considerably if operators are aware of their limitations and apply a systematic approach to their interpretation, as outlined in Chapter 17.

Their diagnostic value will be further enhanced by the increasing use of digital panoramic radiography with all its inherent advantages of image manipulation (see Ch. 16).

Fig. 13.25 Examples of errors owing to patient movement during the exposure cycle.
A Movement of the patient in the vertical plane — distortion of the image in the $\overline{43}$ region (arrowed) caused by opening the mouth. Note that only the part of the patient being imaged at the time of the movement is distorted, the remainder of the film is not affected.
B Continuous shaking movements throughout the cycle.
C Sudden side-to-side movement of the patient in the horizontal plane while the anterior teeth were being imaged causing them to be very blurred.

14 Radiography assessment and localization of unerupted maxillary canines

Radiographic assessment of unerupted maxillary canines

The upper canines are often misplaced and fail to erupt as a result of their long path of eruption, the timing of their eruption and the frequency of upper arch overcrowding. Again, many of the factors that influence the treatment of this anomaly can be obtained from the radiographic assessment, the purpose of which is two-fold:

- To determine the size and shape of the canine and any related disease
- To determine the position of the canine.

Assessment of the canine size and shape and the surrounding tissues

Radiographic views used (see Fig. 14.1)

The usual radiographs used include:

- Periapicals
- Upper standard occlusal
- Dental panoramic tomograph.

Radiographic interpretation

The specific features that need to be examined relate to:

- The crown
- The root
- Surrounding structures.

Note: These views, on their own, do not provide information as to the position of the canines.

The crown

Note in particular:

- Crown size (in relation to the space available in the arch)
- Crown shape
- The presence and severity of resorption
- The presence of any related disease, such as a dentigerous cyst
- The effect on adjacent teeth, such as resorption.

The root

Note in particular:

- Root size
- Root shape
- Stage of development.

Surrounding structures

Note in particular:

- The deciduous canine
  — root length
  — degree of resorption
- The presence of an odontome or supernumerary
- The condition of the surrounding bone.

Assessment of the position of the canine — localization

There are several methods available for localization. They can be used for canines and other unerupted teeth as well as odontomes and supernumeraries.

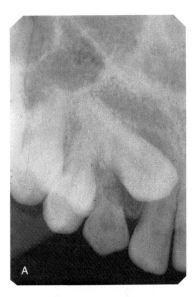

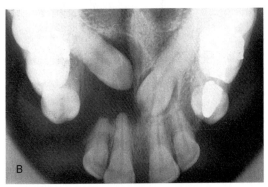

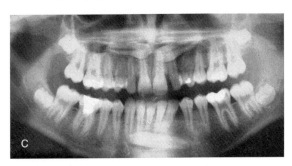

Fig. 14.1 Examples of the radiographs used typically to assess unerupted canines and the surrounding structures.
A Periapical showing unerupted 3/ with retained C/.
B Upper standard occlusal showing both upper canines unerupted, a dentigerous cyst associated with 3/, extensive destruction of the alveolar bone and resorption of /3.
C Dental panoramic tomograph showing unerupted 3/3 and /3.

Although emphasis in this section is on canines, examples of localization of other unerupted developmental anomalies are also shown.

Main localization methods.

- Parallax in the horizontal plane
- Parallax in the vertical plane
- A vertex occlusal
- A true lateral and postero-anterior (PA jaws) (i.e. two views at right angles)
- Stereoscopic views
- Cross-sectional spiral tomography.

The principle of parallax

Parallax is defined as *the apparent displacement of an object because of different positions of the observer.* In other words, if two objects, in two separate planes, are viewed from two different positions, the objects will appear to move in different directions in relation to one another, from one view to the next, as shown in Figure 14.2.

Using the principle of parallax, if two views of an unerupted canine are taken with the X-ray tubehead in two different positions, the resultant radiographs will show a difference in the position of the unerupted canine relative to the incisors, as follows:

- If the canine is **palatally** positioned, it will appear to have moved in the *same* direction as the X-ray tubehead.
- If the canine is **buccally** positioned, it will appear to have moved in the **opposite** direction to the X-ray tubehead.
- If the unerupted canine is in the **same plane** as the incisors, i.e. in the line of the arch, it will appear **not to have moved** at all.

A useful acronym to remember the movements of parallax is SLOB, standing for:

Same
Lingual
Opposite
Buccal.

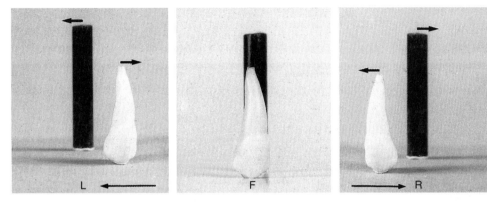

Fig. 14.2 The principle of parallax. Photographs of a small black cylinder positioned behind a tooth. From directly in front (F), the tooth and cylinder are superimposed. With the camera moved to the left (L), the tooth and cylinder are both visible and appear to have moved in different directions. The cylinder, being further away from the camera, appears to have moved in the same direction as the camera, i.e. to the left, while the tooth appears to have moved in the opposite direction. With the camera moved to the right (R) a similar apparent movement of the tooth and cylinder relative to the camera takes place, with the cylinder appearing to have moved to the right and the tooth to the left.

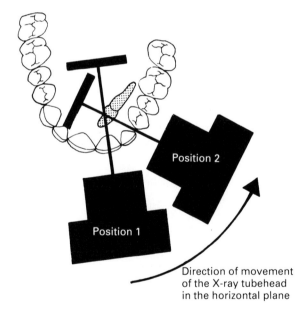

Direction of movement of the X-ray tubehead in the horizontal plane

Fig. 14.3 Diagram showing the two different tubehead positions required for parallax in the horizontal plane: Position (1) centres on the upper central incisor. Position (2) centres on the canine region.

Parallax in the horizontal plane

The movement of the X-ray tubehead is in the horizontal plane, for example:

- 2 periapicals — one centred on the upper central incisor and the other centred on the canine region, as shown in Figure 14.3

- An upper standard occlusal, centred in the midline plus a periapical or an upper oblique occlusal, centred on the canine region.

Examples are shown in Figures 14.4–6.

Note: The advantage of the upper standard occlusal for the initial view is that it shows both sides of the arch and unerupted canines are often bilateral.

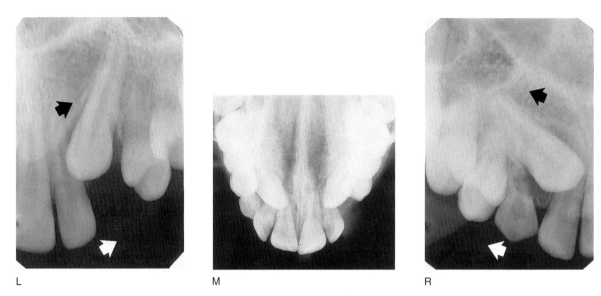

L   M   R

Fig. 14.4 (right) An upper standard occlusal (the mid-line view) and two periapicals centred on the unerupted canines on either side. The teeth can be localized as follows:

1. Examine the midline view radiograph (M), centred on the upper central incisors. The tip of the RIGHT canine appears opposite the root canal of 1/; the tip of the LEFT canine appears opposite the mesial aspect /2.

2. Examine radiograph (R), the periapical centred on the RIGHT canine region (i.e. the X-ray tubehead has been moved distally in the direction of the white arrow). The tip of the canine appears opposite the mesial aspect of 2/. Therefore, it appears to have moved distally in the direction of the black arrow, i.e. in the *same* direction as the X-ray tubehead was moved.

3. Examine radiograph (L), the periapical centred on the LEFT canine region. The tip of the canine appears opposite the root canal of /2. Again both the X-ray tubehead (white arrow) and the canine (black arrow) appear to have moved in the *same* direction.

Thus the crowns of both the right and left canines are *palatally* positioned in relation to the incisors.

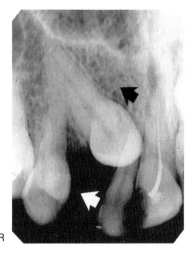
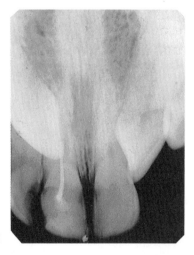

R   M

Fig. 14.5 Two periapicals showing the relative positions of the unerupted 3/ to the incisors — M in the midline and R from the right. The X-ray tubehead (white arrow) and the canine (black arrow) appear to have moved in the *same* direction. The canine is thus palatally positioned.

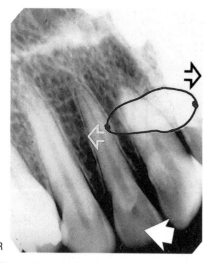

R

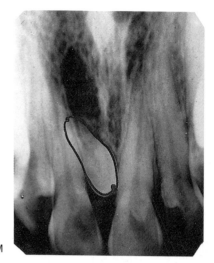

M

Fig. 14.6 Two periapicals showing an unerupted mesiodens. It can be localized as follows:
1. Examine the mid-line radiograph (M). The tip of the mesiodens' crown appears opposite the mesial aspect of /1, while its apex appears opposite the root canal of 1 /.
2. Examine the periapical centred on the RIGHT canine region (R). The tip of the mesiodens crown appears opposite the root canal of /1, while its apex appears opposite the mesial aspect of 2 /.
3. The X-ray tubehead was moved distally in the direction of the large white solid arrow.
4. The crown of the mesiodens appears to have moved mesially (black open arrow), i.e. in the *opposite* direction to the tubehead. It is thus buccally placed.
5. The apex appears to have moved in the *same* direction (white open arrow) as the tubehead and is thus palatally placed.
The mesiodens thus lies across the arch, between the central incisors, with its crown buccally positioned and its apex palatally positioned.

Parallax in the vertical plane

The movement of the X-ray tubehead is in the vertical plane, for example:

* A dental panoramic tomograph — the X-ray beam is aimed upwards at 8° to the horizontal
* An upper standard occlusal — the X-ray beam is aimed downwards at 65°–70° to the horizontal, as shown in Figures 14.7 and 14.8.

Note: This combination of views is used frequently in orthodontics, when patients with unerupted canines are usually assessed. Use of these films to their full potential may obviate the need for further films merely to localize the unerupted canines.

Localization using the vertex occlusal

The vertex occlusal projection was described in detail in Chapter 10. In essence an intraoral cassette is placed in the occlusal plane and the X-ray tubehead is positioned above the patient, in the midline, aiming downwards through the vertex of the skull. The resultant radiograph is a plan view of the maxilla from above. The buccal or palatal position of an unerupted tooth can therefore be determined directly from this one view, as shown in Figure 14.9.

Despite the obvious attraction of this projection, and the ease with which positional assessments can be made, it is not used frequently or recommended because of the inherent disadvantages to the patient including the radiation dose to the eyes, gonads and pituitary gland.

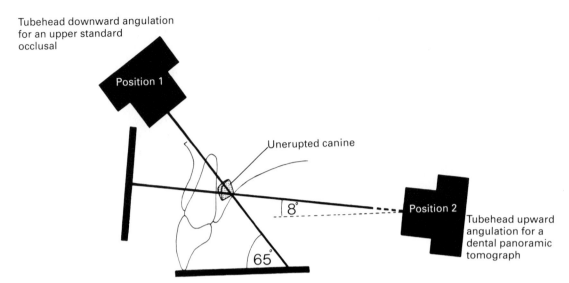

Tubehead downward angulation for an upper standard occlusal

Position 1

Unerupted canine

8°

Position 2

Tubehead upward angulation for a dental panoramic tomograph

65°

Fig. 14.7 Diagram showing the two different tubehead positions when taking a dental panoramic tomograph and an upper standard occlusal, allowing parallax in the vertical plane.

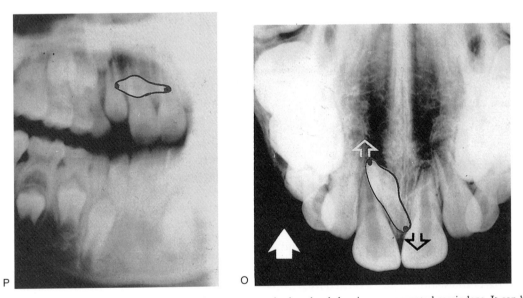

P

O

Fig. 14.8 Part of a dental panoramic tomograph and an upper standard occlusal showing an unerupted mesiodens. It can be localized as follows:

1. Examine the panoramic radiograph (P) taken with the tubehead aimed upwards at 8° to the horizontal. The tip of mesiodens' crown appears opposite the neck of the lateral incisor, while its apex appears opposite the root of /1.
2. Examine the occlusal radiograph (O) taken with the tubehead aimed downwards at 65° to the horizontal. The tip of the mesiodens' crown now appears beyond the apex of 2/, while its apex now appears opposite the crown of /1.
3. The X-ray tubehead has moved vertically upwards from view (P) to view (O) in the direction of the solid white arrow.
4. The crown of the mesiodens appears to have moved in the *same* direction (white open arrow) and is thus palatally placed.
5. The apex of the mesiodens appears to have moved in the *opposite* direction (black open arrow), and is thus buccally placed. The mesiodens thus lies across the arch between the central incisors, with its crown palatally positioned and its apex buccally positioned.

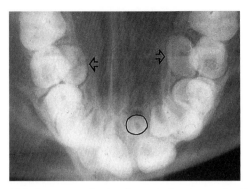

Fig. 14.9 A vertex occlusal radiograph showing a palatally positioned mesiodens (outlined) and palatally positioned premolars (arrowed).

Localization using true lateral and PA jaws radiographs

Localizing unerupted canines using these two skull radiographs was much in vogue in the past. It is seldom used now because although this combination of two films at 90° to each other seems ideal, in practice it is often very difficult to see the unerupted canines satisfactorily and so make an accurate positional assessment.

15 Factors affecting the radiographic image, film faults and quality assurance

This chapter is designed for revision, bringing together and summarizing from earlier chapters the many factors, theoretical and practical, that can affect the radiographic image. It is also designed for quick reference as an aid to fault-finding and correction. Various film faults are illustrated, together with their possible causes. This is followed by a section on quality assurance (QA) and suggested quality control measures.

Image quality

As mentioned in Chapter 1, image quality and the amount of detail shown on a radiograph depend on several factors including:

- Contrast
- Image geometry
- Characteristics of the X-ray beam
- Image sharpness and resolution.

Contrast

Radiographic contrast, i.e. the final visual difference between the various black, white and grey shadows depends on:

- Subject contrast
- Film contrast
- Fog and scatter.

Subject contrast

This is the difference caused by different degrees of attenuation as the X-ray beam is transmitted through different parts of the patient's tissues. It depends upon:

- Differences in tissue thickness
- Differences in tissue density
- Differences in tissue atomic number (photoelectric absorption $\propto Z^3$ (see Ch. 2))
- Quality (voltage (kV)) or penetrating power of the radiation beam.

Film contrast

This is an inherent property of the film itself (see Ch. 5). It determines how the film will respond to the different exposures it receives after the X-ray beam has passed through the patient. Film contrast depends upon four factors:

- The characteristic curve of the film
- Optical density or degree of blackening of the film
- Type of film — direct or indirect action
- Processing.

Fog and scatter

Stray radiation reaching the film either as a result of background fog, or owing to scatter from within the patient, produces unwanted film density (blackening), and thus reduces radiographic contrast.

Image geometry

As mentioned and illustrated in Chapter 1, the geometric accuracy of an image depends upon the position of the X-ray beam, object and film satisfying certain basic geometrical requirements:

- The object and the film should be in contact or as close together as possible
- The object and the film should be parallel to one another
- The X-ray tubehead should be positioned so that the beam meets the object and the film at right angles.

Characteristics of the X-ray beam

The ideal X-ray beam used for imaging should be:

- Sufficiently penetrating to pass through the patient, to a varying degree, and react with the film emulsion to produce good *contrast* between the various black, white and grey shadows (see earlier)
- Parallel, i.e. non-diverging, to prevent magnification of the image (see Ch. 5)
- Produced from a point source to reduce blurring of the image margins and the *penumbra effect* (see Ch. 5).

Image sharpness and resolution

Sharpness is defined as the ability of the X-ray film to define an edge. The main causes of loss of edge definition include:

- Geometric unsharpness including the *penumbra effect* (see above)
- Motion unsharpness, caused by the patient moving during the exposure
- Absorption unsharpness — caused by variation in object shape, e.g. cervical *burn-out* at the neck of a tooth (see Chs. 9 and 18)
- Screen unsharpness, caused by the diffusion and spread of the light emitted from intensifying screens (see Ch. 5)
- Poor resolution. Resolution, or resolving power of the film, is a measure of the film's ability to differentiate between different structures and record separate images of small objects placed very close together, and is determined mainly by characteristics of the film including:
  — type — direct or indirect action
  — speed
  — silver halide emulsion crystal size.
  Resolution is measured in line pairs per mm.

Practical factors influencing image quality

In practical terms, the various factors that can influence overall image quality can be divided into factors related to:

- The X-ray equipment
- The image receptor — film or film/screen combination
- Processing
- The patient
- The operator and radiographic technique.

As a result of all these variables, film faults and alterations in image quality are inevitable. However, since the diagnostic yield from radiography is related directly to the quality of the image, regular checks and monitoring of these variables are essential to achieve and maintain good quality radiographs. It is these checks which form the basis of *quality assurance (QA) programmes* (see later).

Dental nurses need to be able to recognize the cause of the various film faults so that appropriate corrective action can be taken. Repeating a radiograph, without first establishing the cause of the error, may result in the error simply being perpetuated.

Typical film faults

Examples of typical film faults are shown below and summarized later in Table 15.1.

Film too dark (Figs 15.1 and 15.2)

Possible causes

- Overexposure owing to:
  — Faulty X-ray equipment, e.g. timer
  — Incorrect exposure time setting by the operator
- Overdevelopment owing to:
  — Excessive time in the developer solution
  — Developer solution too hot
  — Developer solution too concentrated
- Fogging owing to:
  — Poor storage conditions:
    * Allowing exposure to stray radiation
    * Too warm

— Old film stock i.e. films used after expiry date
— Faulty cassettes allowing ingress of stray light
— Faulty darkroom/processing unit:
  * Allowing leakage of stray light
  * Faulty safe-light
• Thin patient tissues.

Film too pale (Fig. 15.3)

Possible causes

• Underexposure owing to:
  — Faulty X-ray equipment, e.g. timer
  — Incorrect exposure time setting by the operator
  — Failure to keep timer switch depressed throughout the exposure
• Underdevelopment owing to:
  — Inadequate time in the developer solution
  — Developer solution too cold
  — Developer solution too dilute
  — Developer solution exhausted
  — Developer contaminated by fixer
• Excessive thickness of patient's tissues
• Film packet back to front (film also marked).

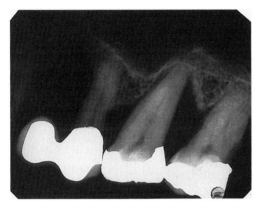

Fig. 15.1 Example of a periapical that is too dark with poor contrast.

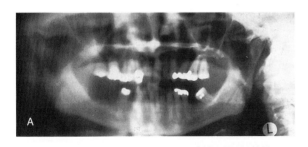

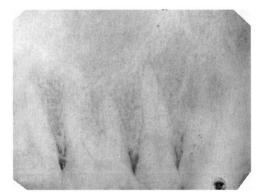

Fig. 15.3 Example of a periapical that is too pale with poor contrast.

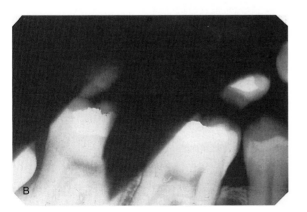

Fig. 15.2 Examples of fogged films. **A** A dental panoramic tomograph taken with a faulty cassette allowing the ingress of light that has fogged (blackened) the RIGHT side of the image. **B** A bitewing that has been fogged in the darkroom by inadvertently exposing the upper part of the film to light. The operator's fingers covered the lower part of the film thus protecting this part of the image.

Film with inadequate or low contrast
(Figs 15.1, 15.2, 15.3)

Possible causes

- Processing error owing to:
  — Underdevelopment (film also pale)
  — Overdevelopment (film also dark)
  — Developer contaminated by fixer
  — Inadequate fixation time
  — Fixer solution exhausted
- Fogging owing to:
  — Poor storage conditions:
    * Allowing exposure to stray radiation
    * Too warm
  — Poor stock control and film used after expiry date
  — Faulty cassettes allowing the ingress of stray light
  — Faulty darkroom/processing unit.

Image unsharp and blurred (Fig. 15.4)

Possible causes

- Movement of the patient during the exposure
- Excessive bending of the film packet during the exposure
- Poor film/screen contact within a cassette
- Film type — image definition is poorer with indirect-action film than with direct-action film

- Speed of intensifying screens — fast screens result in loss of detail
- Overexposure — causing *burn-out* of the edges of a thin object
- Poor positioning in panoramic radiography (see Ch. 13).

Film marked (Fig. 15.5)

Possible causes

- Film packet bent by the operator
- Careless handling of the film in the darkroom resulting in marks caused by:
  — Finger prints
  — Finger nails
  — Bending
  — Static discharge
- Processing errors owing to:
  — Chemical spots
  — Under fixation — residual silver halide emulsion remaining
  — Roller marks
  — Protective black paper becoming stuck to the film
  — Insufficient chemicals to immerse films fully
- Patient biting too hard on the film packet
- Dirty intensifying screens in cassettes.

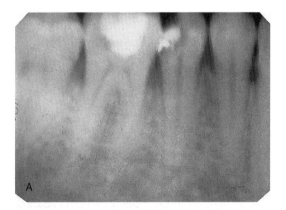 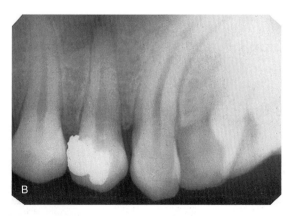

Fig. 15.4 Examples of unsharp and blurred films. **A** As a result of patient movement. **B** As a result of excessive bending of the film packet during the exposure.

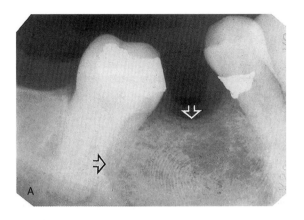

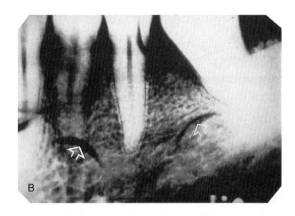

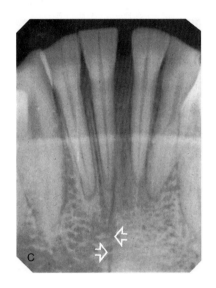

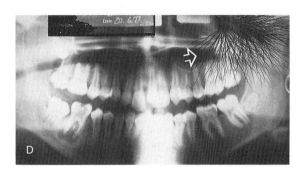

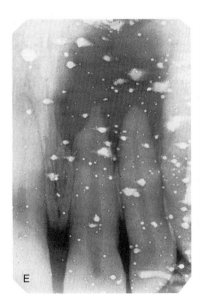

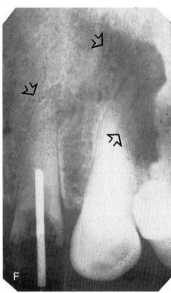

Fig. 15.5 Examples of marked films.

A Finger print impression in the emulsion (arrowed)

B Finger nail marks (arrowed)

C Sharply bent film (arrowed) damaging the emulsion

D Discharge of static electricity (arrowed)

E Fixer splashes on the emulsion before the film was placed in the developer

F Marks (arrowed) caused by residual emulsion remaining following inadequate fixation (these are usually brown).

Table 15.1 Summary of common film quality problems and their possible causes. (Reproduced, with modifications, from Dental Update with kind permission of Prof K. Horner and George Warman Publications.)

Reason for rejection	Possible causes		Remedy to each particular fault
	General	Particular	
Film too dark	Processing fault (overdevelopment)	Developer concentration too high	Dilute or change chemicals
		Development time too long	Adjust as necessary
		Developer temperature too high	Adjust as necessary
	Excessive X-ray exposure	Incorrect exposure setting	Adjust and repeat examination
		Faulty timer on X-ray set	Arrange service and repair of X-ray set
		Thin patient tissues	Decrease exposure and repeat
	Fogged film	Light leak in darkroom	Check and correct
		Faulty safelighting	Inspect safelights visually, coin test, and correct any fault detected
		Old film stock	Discard film
		Poor film storage	Discard film and re-assess storage facilities
		Light leak in cassette	Check hinges and catches and repair or replace if required
Film too pale	Processing fault (underdevelopment)	Overdiluted developer	Change chemicals
		Inadequate development time	Adjust as necessary
		Developer temperature too low	Adjust as necessary
		Exhausted developer	Change chemicals
		Developer contaminated by fixer	Change chemicals
	Inadequate X-ray exposure	Incorrect exposure setting	Adjust and repeat
		Faulty timer on X-ray set	Arrange service and repair of X-ray set
		Excessive thickness of patient's tissues	Increase exposure and repeat
	Technique error	Film back to front	Adjust and repeat
Inadequate or low contrast	Processing fault	Overdevelopment (plus dark films)	Check development and time/temperature relationship
		Underdevelopment (plus pale films)	As above
		Developer contaminated by fixer (films opaque; milky sheen)	Change chemicals
		Inadequate fixation time (films opaque; milky sheen)	Adjust as necessary
		Fixer exhausted (films opaque; milky sheen)	Change fixer solution
	Fogged film	See above	See above

Unsharp image	Technique error	Patient movement	Assess and instruct patient carefully
		Excessive bending of the film packet during exposure	Adjust and repeat
		Poor patient positioning (in panoramic radiography)	Greater care in positioning and full use of positioning aids
	Cassette error	Poor film/screen contact	Check cassette and repair or replace if necessary
		Incorrect intensifying screen speed	Change screens
Film marked	Excessive X-ray exposure	Incorrect exposure setting for thin object causing *burn-out*	Decrease exposure setting and repeat
	Handling fault	Film packet bent	Careful handling
		Careless handling in darkroom	As above
	Processing fault	Chemical spots	Careful chemical handling
		Insufficient chemicals to allow full immersion of film	Check chemical tanks and adjust
		Automatic roller marks	Clean processor
		Patient biting too hard on the film	Instruct patient correctly and repeat
		Dirt on intensifying screens	Clean screens regularly
Poor positioning	Film packet incorrectly positioned	Film back to front (plus pale film)	Use film holders for intraoral radiography when possible
		Not covering area of interest	As above
		Film used twice (plus dark film)	Greater care in film handling
	X-ray tubehead incorrectly positioned	Too steep an angle producing foreshortening	Use beam-aiming devices when possible
		Too shallow an angle producing elongation	As above
	Patient incorrectly positioned	Patient incorrectly placed (in panoramic unit)	Greater care in positioning and full use of positioning aids

Operator positioning errors (Fig. 15.6)

Typical positioning faults

Intraoral radiographic positioning faults include:

- Incorrect placement of the X-ray tubehead producing:
  — Elongation
  — Foreshortening
  — Superimposition/overlapping
  — *Coning off* or *cone cutting*

- Incorrect placement of the film packet:
  — Back to front, image of the lead foil evident (film also too pale)
  — Inadvertently used twice, double exposure (film also too dark)
  — Not covering the area of interest.

Note: Positioning errors specific to dental panoramic tomographs are shown in Chapter 3.

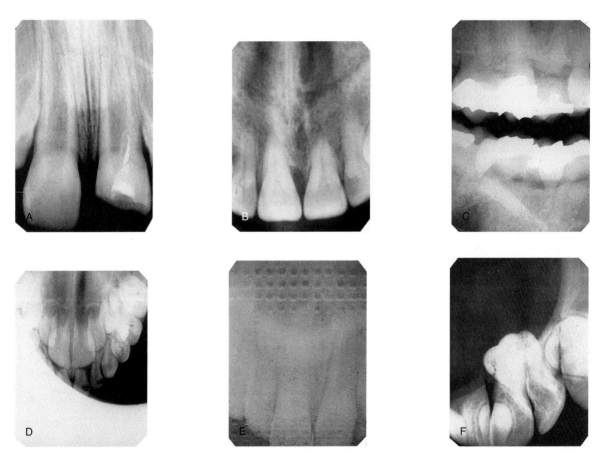

Fig. 15.6 Examples of operator positioning errors.
A Elongated image — the vertical angulation of the X-ray tubehead was too shallow.
B Foreshortened image — the vertical angulation of the X-ray tubehead was too steep.
C Superimposition/overlapping of adjacent structures — the horizontal angulation of the X-ray tubehead was incorrect.
D *Coning off* or *cone cutting* — the X-ray tubehead was placed too far posteriorly so that the anterior part of film was not exposed.
E Pattern from the lead foil is evident — the film packet was placed back to front in the mouth.
F Double exposure — the same film packet was used for two different projections.

Quality assurance in dental radiology

The World Health Organization has defined radiographic quality assurance (QA) programmes as '... an organised effort by the staff operating a facility to ensure that the diagnostic images produced by the facility are of sufficiently high quality so that they consistently provide adequate diagnostic information at the lowest possible cost and with the least possible exposure of the patient to radiation'.

Quality control measures are therefore as essential in a general dental practice *facility*, as they are in a specialized radiography department. This importance of **quality** is acknowledged in the UK in the Ionising Radiations Regulations 1999 (see Ch. 6) which make quality assurance in dental radiography a mandatory requirement. A section in the 2001 *Guidance Notes for Dental Practitioners on the Safe Use of X-ray Equipment* is devoted to quality assurance and should be regarded as essential reading for dental nurses. This chapter is based broadly on the recommendations in the 2001 *Guidance Notes*.

Terminology

The main terms in quality procedures include:

- *Quality control* — the specific measures for ensuring and verifying the quality of the radiographs produced.
- *Quality assurance* — the arrangements to ensure that the quality control procedures are effective and that they lead to relevant change and improvement.
- *Quality audit* — the process of external reassurance and assessment that quality control and quality assurance mechanisms are satisfactory and that they work effectively.

Quality assurance programme

A basic principle of quality assurance is that, within the overall QA programme, all necessary procedures should be laid down in writing and in particular:

- Implementation should be the responsibility of a named person
- Frequency of operations should be defined
- The content of the essential supporting records should be defined and the frequency for the formal checking of such records.

As stated in the 2001 *Guidance Notes* and implied by the WHO definition, a well-designed QA programme should be comprehensive but inexpensive to operate and maintain. The standards should be well researched but once laid down would be expected to require only infrequent verification or modification. The procedures should amount to little more than 'written down common sense'. The aims of these programmes can be summarized as follows:

- To produce diagnostic radiographs of consistently high standard
- To reduce the number of repeat radiographs
- To determine all sources of error to allow their correction
- To increase efficiency
- To reduce costs
- To ensure that radiation doses to patients and staff are kept as low as reasonably practicable (ALARP).

Quality control procedures

The essential quality control procedures relate to:

- Image quality and film reject analysis
- Patient dose and X-ray equipment
- Darkroom, image receptors and processing
- Working procedures
- Staff training and updating
- Audits.

Image quality and film reject analysis

Image quality assessment is an important test of the entire QA programme. Hence the need for clinicians to be aware of all the various factors, outlined earlier, that affect image quality and to monitor it on a regular basis. This assessment should include:

- A day-to-day comparison of the quality of every radiograph to a high standard reference film positioned permanently on the viewing screen and an investigation of any significant deterioration in quality.
- A formal analysis of film quality, either retrospective or prospective, approximately every 6 months. The *Guidance Notes* recommend that the simple three-point subjective rating scale shown in Table 15.2, originally suggested by the NRPB/RCR in their 1994 *Guidelines*, be used for dental radiography.
- Based on these quality ratings, performance targets can be set. Suitable targets recommended in the *Guidance Notes* are shown in Table 15.3 with the advice that practices should aim to achieve these targets within 3 years of implementing the QA programme. The 'interim targets' should be regarded as the minimum achievable standard in the shorter term.
- Analysis of all unacceptable films given a rating of 3, sometimes referred to as *film reject analysis* (see below).

Film reject analysis

This is a simple method of identifying all film faults and sources of error and amounts to a *register of reject radiographs*. To do this, it is necessary to collect all rejected (grade 3) radiographs and record:

Table 15.2 Subjective quality rating of radiographs originally from the NRPB/RCR *Guidelines on Radiology Standards in Primary Dental Care* 1994 and used in the 2001 *Guidance Notes*.

Rating	Quality	Basis
1	Excellent	No errors of exposure, positioning or processing
2	Diagnostically acceptable	Some errors of exposure, positioning or processing, but which do not detract from the diagnostic utility of the radiograph
3	Unacceptable	Errors of exposure, positioning or processing which render the radiograph unacceptable

Table 15.3 Minimum and interim targets for radiographic quality from the 2001 *Guidance Notes*

	Percentage of radiographs taken	
Rating	Target	Interim target
1	Not less than 70%	Not less than 50%
2	Not greater than 20%	Not less than 40%
3	Not greater than 10%	Not greater than 10%

- Date
- Nature of the film fault/error, as shown earlier, e.g.:
  a. Film too dark
  b. Film too pale
  c. Low or poor contrast
  d. Unsharp image
  e. Poor positioning
- Known or suspected cause of the error or fault and corrective action taken (see Table 15.1)
- Number of repeat radiographs (if taken)
- Total number of radiographs taken during the same time period. This allows the percentage of faulty films to be calculated.

Regular review of film reject analysis records is an invaluable aid for identifying a range of problems, including a need for equipment maintenance, additional staff training as well as processing faults that could otherwise cause unnecessary radiation exposure of patients and staff.

Patient dose and X-ray equipment

One of the aims of QA stated earlier is to ensure that radiation doses are kept as low as reasonably practicable. X-ray equipment must comply with current Recommendations (see Ch. 6). Dental nurses should familiarise themselves with the equipment and the supporting documentation. Important points to note include:

- The initial *critical examination and report* — carried out by the installer
- The *acceptance test* — carried out by the radiation protection adviser before equipment is brought into clinical use and includes measurement of patient dose

- A *re-examination report* following any relocation, repair or modification of equipment that may have radiation protection implications
- Day-to-day checks of important features that could affect radiation protection including:
  — correct functioning of warning lights and audible alarms
  — correct operation of safety devices
  — satisfactory performance of the counterbalance for maintaining the correct position of the tubehead
- Written records and an equipment log should be maintained and include:
  — all installer's formal written reports describing the checks made, the results obtained and action taken
  — results of all equipment checks in chronological order
  — details of all routine or special maintenance
- The Ionizing Radiation (Medical Exposure) Regulations 2000 require that an up-to-date inventory of each item of X-ray equipment is maintained, and available, at each practice and contains:
  — name of the manufacturer
  — model number
  — serial number or other unique identifier
  — year of manufacture
  — year of installation.

Darkroom, image receptors and processing

Darkroom

The QA programme should include instructions on all the regular checks that should be made, and how frequently, with all results recorded in a log. Important areas include:

- General cleanliness (daily), but particularly of work surfaces and film hangers (if used)
- Light-tightness (yearly), by standing in the darkroom in total darkness with the door closed and safelights switched off and visually inspecting for light leakage
- Safelights (yearly), to ensure that these do not cause fogging of films. Checks are required on:
  — Type of filter — this should be compatible with the colour sensitivity of film used, i.e. blue, green or ultraviolet (see Ch. 5)
  — Condition of filters — scratched filters should be replaced
  — Wattage of the bulb — ideally it should be no more than 25 W
  — Their distance from the work surface — ideally they should be at least 1.2 m (4 ft) away
  — Overall safety (i.e. their fogging effect on film) — the simple quality control measure for doing this is known as the *coin test*:
  1. Expose a piece of screen film in a cassette to a very small even exposure of X-rays (so-called *flash* exposure) to make the emulsion ultra-sensitive to subsequent light exposure
  2. In the darkroom, remove the film from the cassette and place on the worksurface underneath the turned-off safelight
  3. Place a series of coins (e.g. seven) in a row on the film and cover them all with a piece of card
  4. Turn on the safelight and then slide the card to reveal the first coin and leave for approximately 30 seconds
  5. Slide the card along to reveal the second coin and leave again for approximately 30 seconds
  6. Repeat until all the coins have been revealed
  7. Process the film in the normal way.

A simulated result is shown in Figure 15.7. Fogging (blackening) of the film owing to the safelight will then be obvious when compared to the clear area protected by the coin. The part of the film adjacent to the first coin will have been exposed to the safelight for the longest time and will be the darkest. In practice, the normal film-handling time under the safelight can be measured and the effect of safelight fogging established.

Note. The *coin test* can also be used to assess the amount of light transmission through the safety glass of automatic processors by performing the test within the processor under the safety glass under normal daylight loading conditions.

Image receptors

The QA programme requires written information, usually obtained from the suppliers, on film speed, expiry date and storage conditions as well as details regarding the maintenance and cleaning instructions of cassettes and/or digital image receptors. Typical requirement could include:

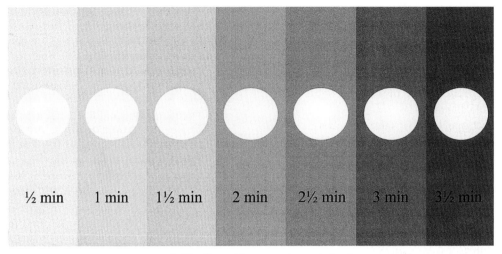

½ min 1 min 1½ min 2 min 2½ min 3 min 3½ min

Fig. 15.7 A simulated coin test result. The film, with seven coins on it, has been gradually uncovered every 30 seconds. The coin-covered part of the film remains white while the surrounding film is blackened or fogged. The longer the film is exposed to the safelight the darker it becomes. (Kindly provided by Mr N. Drage.)

X-ray film *requires:*

- Ideal storage conditions — cool, dry and away from all sources of ionizing radiation — as recommended by the manufacturers
- Strict stock control with records to ensure usage before the expiry date
- Careful handling.

Cassettes *require:*

- Regular cleaning of intensifying screens with a proprietary cleaner
- Regular checks for light-tightness, as follows:
  1. Load a cassette with an unexposed film and place the cassette on a window sill in the daylight for a few minutes
  2. Process the film — any ingress of light will have fogged (darkened) the film (see Fig. 15.8(i))
- Regular checks for film/screen contact, as follows:
  1. Load a cassette with an unexposed film and a similar sized piece of graph paper
  2. Expose the cassette to X-rays using a very short exposure time
  3. Process the film — any areas of poor film/screen contact will be demonstrated by loss of definition of the image of the graph paper (see Fig. 15.8(ii))

- A simple method of identification of films taken in similar looking cassettes, e.g. a Letraset letter on one screen.

Digital phosphor storage plates *require:*

- Regular cleaning
- Regular visual checks for scratches or other defects.

Processing

The QA programme should contain written instructions about each of the following:

Chemical solutions. These should be:

- Always made up to the manufacturers' instructions taking special precautions to avoid even trace amounts of contamination of the developer by the fixer, e.g. always fill the fixer tank first so that any splashes into the developer tank can be washed away **before** pouring in the developer
- Always at the correct temperature
- Changed or replenished regularly — ideally every 2 weeks — and records should be kept to control and validate these changes
- Monitored for deterioration. This can be done easily using radiographs of a *step-wedge phantom*:

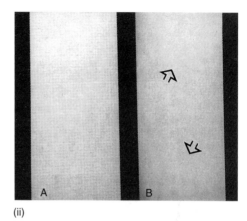

(ii)

Fig. 15.8(ii) Examples of the radiographs following the graph paper test for film/screen contact. **A** Good film/screen contact—the fine detail of the graph paper is evident over the whole film. **B** Poor film/screen contact—note the loss of detail in several areas.

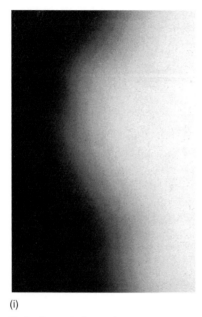

(i)

Fig. 15.8(i) Radiograph from a faulty cassette being checked for light-tightness. The light that has got into the cassette has blackened one side of the film.

1. Make a simple step-wedge phantom using the lead foil from inside intra-oral film packets, as shown in Figure 15.9(i)
2. Radiograph the step-wedge using known exposure factors
3. Process the film in **fresh** solutions to produce a *standard reference film*
4. Repeat, using the same exposure factors, every day as the solutions become exhausted
5. Compare each day's film with the standard reference film to determine objectively any decrease in blackening of the processed film which would indicate deterioration of the developer (see Fig. 15.9(ii))
6. Record the results.

Processing equipment

- Manual processing requires the use of accurate timers, thermometers and immersion heaters. Instructions on their proper use should be provided.
- Automatic processors require regular replenishment of chemical solutions and regular cleaning, especially of the rollers. All cleaning procedures should be written down including how often they should be carried out.

- Record log confirming that all cleaning procedures have been carried out should be kept.

Working procedures

These include:

- *Local rules* — required in the UK under the Ionising Radiations Regulations 1999 (see Ch. 6). These rules should contain the procedural and operational elements that are essential to the safe use of X-ray equipment, including guidance on exposure times, and as such should contain much of what is relevant to the maintenance of good standards in QA.
- *Employers' written procedures* — required in the UK under the Ionising Radiation (Medical Exposure) Regulations 2000 (see Ch. 6).
- *Operational procedures or systems of work* — these include written procedures that provide for all actions that indirectly affect radiation safety and diagnostic quality, e.g. instructions for the correct preparation and subsequent use of processing chemicals (as explained earlier).
- *Procedures log* — the QA programme should include the maintenance of a procedures log to record the existence of appropriate *Local Rules* and *Employers' Written Procedures*, together with a record of each occasion on which they are reviewed or modified (ideally every 12 months).

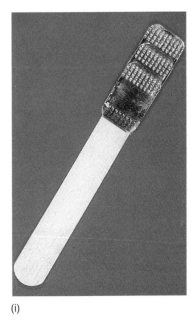

(i)

Fig. 15.9(i) A simple step-wedge phantom constructed using pieces of lead foil taped to a tongue spatula.

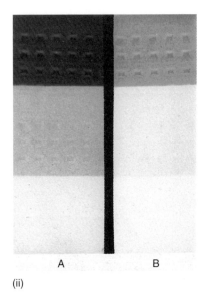

A   B

(ii)

Fig. 15.9(ii) **A** The *standard reference* film of the step-wedge phantom on DAY ONE processed using newly made-up chemical solutions. **B** Test film processed in chemical solutions 1 week old — note the reduced amount of blackening of the second film owing to the weakened action of the developer.

Staff training and updating

As mentioned in Chapter 6, it is a legal requirement under the Ionising Radiation (Medical Exposure) Regulations 2000 that all practitioners and operators (dental nurses) are adequately trained and that continuing professional development (CPD) is undertaken. The details of the training required in the UK are given in Chapter 6. The QA programme should incorporate a register of all staff involved with any aspect of radiography and should include the following information:

* Name
* Responsibility
* Date, nature and details of training received
* Recommended date for a review of training needs.

Audits

Each procedure within the QA programme will include a requirement for written records to be made by the responsible person at varying intervals. In addition, the person with overall responsibility for the QA programme should check the full programme at intervals not exceeding 12 months.

This is an essential feature of demonstrating effective implementation of the programme. Clinical audits may include:

* The QA programme and associated records
* The justification and authorisation of radiographs
* The appropriateness of requests/investigations
* The clinical evaluation of radiographs.

Footnote

The requirement for quality assurance and quality control measures in general dental practice applies equally to specialized radiography departments. However, in view of the cost implications, the expensive, sophisticated equipment available for precise quality assurance measurements and accurate monitoring in X-ray departments are often inappropriate to general practice. The practical suggestions in this chapter, based on the 2001 *Guidance Notes*, are designed to satisfy the WHO definition by bringing an element of objectivity to quality assurance in practice, but at the same time being simple, easily done and inexpensive.

16 Digital radiography

Introduction

Digital images are acquired either *directly* — using a sensor or imaging plate replacing conventional film (as described below) or *indirectly* — by scanning and digitizing a film-captured image.

Direct digital imaging systems are divided into two types:

- Real time or *corded*
- Photostimulable phosphor storage plate or *cordless*.

Real-time or corded systems

These systems employ conventional X-ray-generating equipment but conventional film is replaced by either a *CCD (charge coupled device)* or a *CMOS (complementary metal oxide semiconductor)* sensor which is connected to the computer via a cable (or *cord*). The X-ray photons that reach the sensor are converted to light, by an intensifying or scintillation screen, which is picked by the CCD/CMOS and converted into an electrical charge which, once relayed to the computer, produces an almost instantaneous digital image on the monitor (hence the term *real time*). Several dental systems are now available; a well-known example is Trophy's Radiovisiography® (RVG) (see Fig. 16.1).

Different sized intraoral, as well as panoramic, sensors are produced, as shown in Figure 16.2.

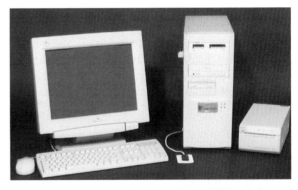

Fig. 16.1 The Trophy Radiovisiography® (RVG) real-time digital imaging system where the CCD sensor is connected directly to the computer.

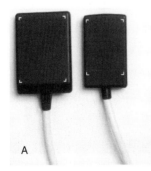

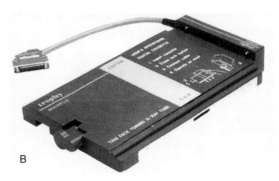

Fig. 16.2 A Two intraoral Trophy RVG CCD sensors. **B** Trophy Digipan® panoramic CCD sensor.

Specially designed intraoral sensor holders (with and without beam-aiming devices), similar to those used for conventional film (see Ch. 8), have been developed as shown in Figure 16.3. When used clinically, the sensors need to be covered with a protective plastic barrier envelope for infection control purposes (see Ch. 7, Fig. 7.4).

Photostimulable phosphor imaging or cordless systems

These systems employ re-usable *photostimulable phosphor imaging plates (PSPP)* instead of film. The plates contain a layer of barium fluorohalide phosphor, as shown in Figure 16.4.

The phosphor layer absorbs and stores the X-ray energy that has not been attenuated by the patient. The image plate is then placed in a reader where it is scanned by a laser beam. The stored X-ray energy in the phosphor layer is released as light which is detected by a photomultiplier. From here the information is relayed to the computer and displayed as a digital image on the monitor. The time taken to read the plate depends on the particular system being used, and on the size of the plate, but usually varies between approximately 1 and 5 minutes. Again, several dental systems are available, including Soredex's Digora® fmx and the Gendex® DenOptix™ (see Fig. 16.5).

A range of intraoral plate sizes is available with the DenOptix® system, identical in size to conventional periapical and occlusal film packets. Extraoral plates for panoramic and skull radiography are also available, as shown in Figure 16.6.

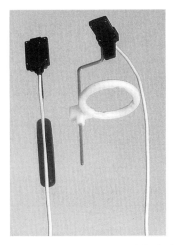

Fig. 16.3 Intraoral CCD sensors in specially designed and adapted holders for clinical use.

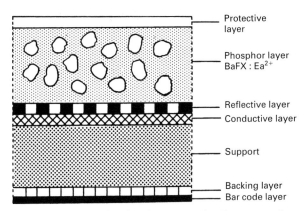

Protective layer

Phosphor layer BaFX : Ea^{2+}

Reflective layer
Conductive layer

Support

Backing layer
Bar code layer

Fig. 16.4 Diagram showing the cross-sectional structure of a typical phosphor imaging plate.

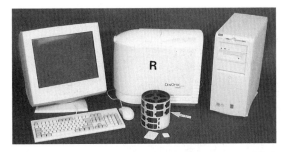

Fig. 16.5 The DenOptix™ photostimulable phosphor digital imaging system. The exposed plates are attached to the drum (arrowed) which is then inserted into the reader (R).

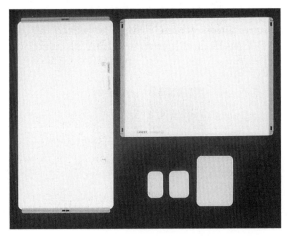

Fig. 16.6 The different sized DenOptix™ plates for panoramic, skull and intraoral radiography.

Radiographic techniques are identical to those using conventional film. The intraoral plates are inserted into protective barrier envelopes (see Fig. 16.7) and can then be used in conventional film holders. The extraoral plates are placed in conventional cassettes after the intensifying screens have been removed.

Theory

As computers deal with numbers and not pictures, a radiographic image within a computer is represented as a sequence of numbers. This image may be considered as a grid or matrix of tiny boxes or pixels. Each pixel has an x and y coordinate and is rendered as a numbered sequence dependent on the amount of X-ray attenuation in each box. Each number, and hence each pixel, is then assigned an appropriate shade of grey. The number and size of the pixels, together with the number of shades of grey available, determine

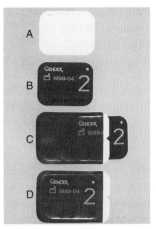

Fig. 16.7 A The white imaging side of a DenOptix™ phosphor plate. **B** The reverse side of the plate. **C** The plate being inserted into the protective barrier envelope — note the reverse side of the plate is visible through the clear side of the envelope. **D** The plate in the envelope ready for clinical use.

the amount of information in an image, the size of the image file and the resolution of the final image (see Fig. 16.8). The resolution (in line pairs per

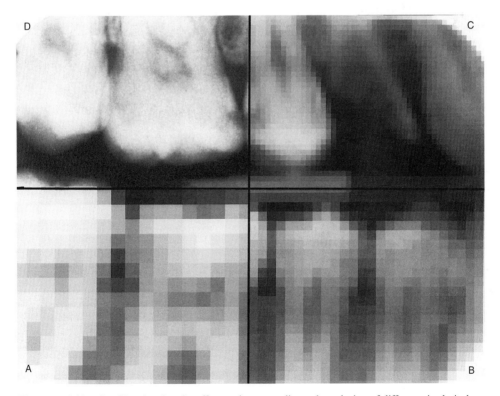

Fig. 16.8 A bitewing film showing the effect on image quality and resolution of different sized pixels gradually reducing from **A** to **D**.

mm) of modern digital images on the screen is comparable with, and may be better than, film (see Ch. 5).

The picture can be changed by giving the pixels different numbers. The coordinates of pixels may be changed or swapped, allowing different parts of the image to be moved around. The shades of grey may be altered or different colours used. These variables are the basis for image processing or manipulation. Despite being able to alter the final image, the computer cannot provide any additional real information to that contained in the original image. It should be remembered that although enhancement may make images look aesthetically more pleasing (see Fig. 16.9), it may also cause clinical information to be lost and diagnoses compromised.

Advantages over conventional film-based radiography

- Lower dose of radiation required as both types of digital image receptors are much more efficient at recording photon energy than conventional films
- No need for conventional processing, thus avoiding all processing film faults (see Ch. 15) and the hazards associated with handling the chemical solutions
- Easy storage and archiving of patient information and incorporation into patient records
- Easy transfer of images electronically (teleradiology)
- Image enhancement and processing. Current software packages allow several image enhancement techniques including:
  — inversion (reversal)
  — alteration in contrast
  — embossing or pseudo 3-D
  — magnification
  — automated measurement
  — pseudocolourization.

These are shown on Figure 16.9.

Disadvantages

- Expensive, especially panoramic systems
- Long-term storage of the images although this should be solved by saving them on CD-ROM
- Digital image security and the need to back up data
- The connecting cable (or cord) can make intraoral placement of these system's sensors difficult
- Loss of image quality and resolution on the hard copy print-out when using thermal, laser or ink-jet printers
- Image manipulation can be time-consuming and misleading to the inexperienced
- While manufacturers provide safeguards to any tampering with original images within their own software, it is relatively easy to access these images using cheap third-party software and then to change them, as shown in Figure 16.9.

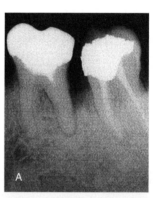

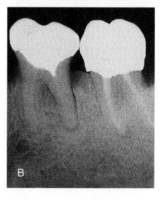

Fig. 16.9 An example of image alteration using third-party software. **A** Original image — note the bony defect between the /6 and /7, the lack of contact point and the restoration in /7. **B** After digital manipulation and no clinical treatment. (Kindly provided by Mr N. Drage.)

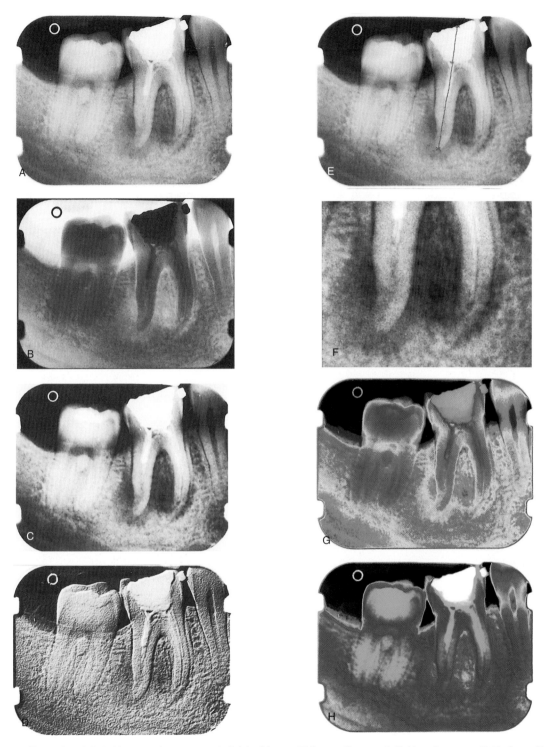

Fig. 16.10 Examples of digital image enhancement: **A** Original image. **B** Inverted/reversed. **C** Altered contrast. **D** Embossed/pseudo 3-D. **E** Automated measurement. **F** Magnified. **G** and **H** Pseudo-coloured. (Kindly provided by Mr N. Drage.)

Important points to note

- Computed or digital radiography is undoubtedly the promising imaging modality of the future, although it may take several years before the total filmless dental practice becomes reality.

- Conventional radiographic film image quality is dependent on three main variables: geometric accuracy, exposure factors and chemical processing (see Ch. 15). Digital imaging eliminates chemical processing and can compensate for some exposure variation, but it still requires the accurate practical taking of the image. The ideal geometrical relationship between image receptor, object and X-ray beam outlined in Chapter 1 and shown in Figure 1.10, still applies — hence the need for sensor holders and beam-aiming devices.

- Computed or digital radiographic images are two-dimensional representations of three-dimensional objects and therefore share this important, inherent limitation with conventional radiographs.

- Digital panoramics are still tomographic slices with their inherent disadvantages (see Ch. 13).

Radiology

Part 5

17 Introduction to radiological interpretation

Interpretation of radiographs can be regarded as an unravelling process — uncovering all the information contained within the black, white and grey radiographic images. The main objectives are:

- To identify the presence or absence of disease
- To provide information on the nature and extent of the disease
- To enable the formation of a differential diagnosis.

To achieve these objectives and maximize the diagnostic yield, interpretation should be carried out under specified conditions, following ordered, systematic guidelines.

Unfortunately, interpretation is often limited to a cursory glance under totally inappropriate conditions. It is easy to fall victim to the problems and pitfalls produced by *spot diagnosis* and *tunnel vision*. This is in spite of knowing that in most cases radiographs are the main diagnostic aid.

This chapter provides an introductory approach to how radiographs should be interpreted, specifying the viewing conditions required and suggesting systematic guidelines.

Essential requirements for interpretation

The essential requirements for interpreting dental radiographs can be summarized as follows:

- Optimum viewing conditions
- Understanding the nature and limitations of the black, white and grey radiographic image
- Knowledge of what the radiographs used in dentistry should look like, so a critical assessment of individual film quality can be made
- Detailed knowledge of the range of radiographic appearances of normal anatomical structures
- Detailed knowledge of the radiographic appearances of the pathological conditions affecting the head and neck
- A systematic approach to viewing the entire radiograph and to viewing and describing specific lesions
- Access to previous films for comparison.

Optimum viewing conditions

These include:

- An even, uniform, bright light viewing screen (preferably of variable intensity to allow viewing of films of different densities) (see Fig. 17.1)
- A quiet, darkened viewing room
- The area around the radiograph should be masked by a dark surround so that light passes only through the film
- Use of a magnifying glass to allow fine detail to be seen more clearly on intraoral films
- The radiographs should be dry.

These ideal viewing conditions give the observer the best chance of perceiving all the detail contained within the radiographic image. With many simultaneous external stimuli, such as extraneous light and inadequate viewing conditions, the amount of information obtained from the radiograph is reduced (see Fig. 17.2). Radiographs should be viewed once they have dried as films still wet from processing may show some distortion of the image.

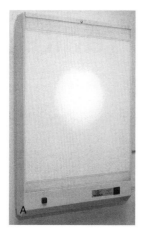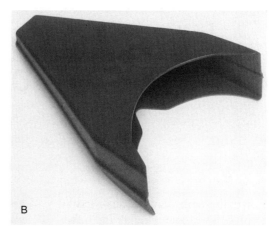

Fig. 17.1A Wardray viewing box incorporating an additional central bright-light source for viewing over-exposed dark films. **B** The SDI X-ray reader — an extraneous light excluding intraoral film viewer with built-in magnification.

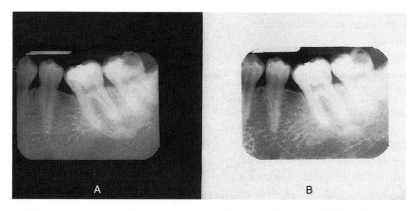

Fig. 17.2 The effect of different viewing conditions on the same periapical radiograph. **A** With a black surround. **B** With a white surround. Note the increased detail visible in **A**, particularly around the molar teeth.

The nature and limitations of the radiographic image

The importance of understanding the nature and limitations of the radiographic image was explained in Chapter 1. (Revision of Chapter 1 is recommended to remember the architect's house and the problems of perception.) To reiterate, the final image was described as 'a two-dimensional picture made up of a variety of black, white and grey superimposed shadows' — a *shadowgraph*.

Critical assessment of radiographic quality

To be able to assess and interpret any radiograph correctly, observers have to know what that radiograph should look like and which structures should be shown. It is for this reason that the chapters on radiography included:

1. WHY each projection was taken
2. HOW the projections were taken
3. WHAT the resultant radiographs should look like and which anatomical features they showed.

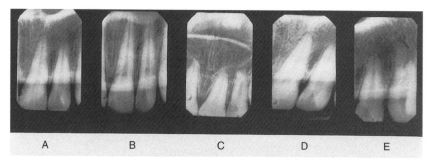

Fig. 17.3 Examples of how variations in radiographic technique can alter the images produced of the same object. **A** Correct projection. **B** Incorrect vertical angulation producing an elongated image. **C** Incorrect vertical angulation producing a foreshortened image. **D** and **E** Incorrect horizontal angulations producing distorted images.

With this practical knowledge of radiography, dental nurses are in a position to make an *overall critical assessment* of individual films.

The practical factors that can influence *image quality* were discussed in Chapter 15, and included:

- The X-ray equipment
- The image receptor-film or film/screen combination
- Processing
- The patient
- The operator and radiographic technique.

A critical assessment of radiographs can be made by combining these factors and by asking a series of questions about the final image. These questions relate to:

- Radiographic technique
- Exposure factors and film density
- Processing.

Here are some typical examples.

Technique (see Fig. 17.3)

- Which technique has been used?
- How were the patient, film and X-ray tubehead positioned?
- Is this a good example of this particular radiographic projection?
- How much distortion is present?
- Is the image foreshortened or elongated?
- Is there any rotation or asymmetry?
- How good are the image resolution and sharpness?
- Has the film been fogged?
- Which artefactual shadows are present?
- How do these technique variables alter the final radiographic image?

Exposure factors (see Fig. 17.4)

- Is the radiograph correctly exposed for the specific reason it was requested?
- Is it too dark and so possibly overexposed?
- Is it too light/pale and so possibly underexposed?
- How good is the contrast?
- What effect will exposure factor variation have on the zone under investigation?

Processing

- Is the radiograph correctly processed?
- Is it too dark and so possibly overdeveloped?
- Is it too pale and so possibly underdeveloped?
- Is it dirty with emulsion still present and so underfixed?
- Is the film wet or dry?

With experience, this critical assessment of quality is not a lengthy procedure but it is one that should never be overlooked. A poor quality radiograph is a poor diagnostic aid and sometimes may be of no diagnostic value at all.

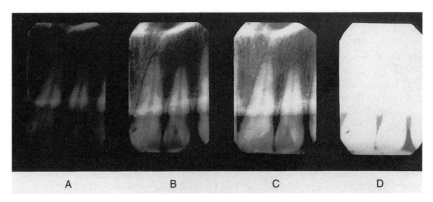

Fig. 17.4 Examples of how variations in exposure factors can alter the image quality of the same object. **A** Overexposed. **B** Slightly overexposed. **C** Correctly exposed. **D** Underexposed.

Detailed knowledge of normal anatomy

A detailed knowledge of the radiographic appearances of **normal** anatomical structures is necessary if observers are to be able to recognize the **abnormal** appearances of the many diseases that affect the jaws.

Not only is a comprehensive knowledge of hard and soft tissue anatomy required but also a knowledge of:

- The type of radiograph being interpreted (e.g. conventional radiograph or tomograph)
- The position of the patient, film and X-ray tubehead.

Only with **all** this information can observers appreciate how the various normal anatomical structures, through which the X-ray beam has passed, will appear on any particular radiograph.

Detailed knowledge of pathological conditions

Radiological interpretation depends on recognition of the typical patterns and appearances of different diseases. The more important appearances,

that dental nurses should be able to recognize, are described in Chapters 18–22.

Systematic approach

A systematic approach to viewing radiographs is necessary to ensure that no relevant information is missed. This systematic approach should apply to:

- The entire radiograph
- Specific lesions.

The entire radiograph

Any systematic approach will suffice as long as it is logical, ordered and thorough. Several suggested sequences are described in later chapters. By way of an example, a suggested systematic approach to the overall interpretation of dental panoramic tomographs (see Ch. 13) is shown in Figure 17.5.

This type of ordered sequential viewing of radiographs requires discipline on the part of the observer. It is easy to be sidetracked by noticing something unusual or abnormal, thus forgetting the remainder of the radiograph.

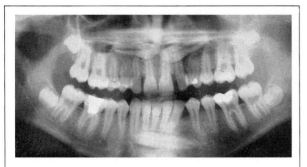

GENERAL OVERVIEW OF THE ENTIRE FILM
1. Note the chronological and development age of the patient.
2. Trace the outline of all normal anatomical shadows and compare their shape and radiodensity.

THE TEETH
3. Note particularly:
   a. The number of teeth present
   b. Stage of development
   c. Position
   d. Condition of the crowns
      (i) Caries
      (ii) Restorations
   e. Condition of the roots
      (i) Length
      (ii) Fillings
      (iii) Resorption
      (iv) Crown/root ratio.

THE APICAL TISSUES
4. Note particularly:
   a. The integrity of lamina dura
   b. Any radiolucencies or opacities associated with the apices.

THE PERIODONTAL TISSUES
5. Note particularly:
   a. The width of the periodontal ligament
   b. The level and quality of crestal bone
   c. Any vertical or horizontal bone loss
   d. Any furcation involvements
   e. Any calculus deposits.

THE BODY AND RAMUS OF THE MANDIBLE
6. Note:
   a. Shape
   b. Outline
   c. Thickness of the lower border
   d. Trabeculae pattern
   e. Any radiolucent or radiopaque areas
   f. Shape of the condylar heads.

OTHER STRUCTURES
7. These include:
   a. The antra, note:
      (i) The outline of the floor, and anterior and posterior walls
      (ii) Radiodensity
   b. Nasal cavity
   c. Styloid processes.

Fig. 17.5 An example of a dental panoramic tomograph and a suggested systematic sequence for viewing this type of film.

Specific lesions

A systematic description of a lesion should include its:

- Site or anatomical position
- Size
- Shape
- Outline/edge or periphery
- Relative radiodensity and internal structure
- Effect on adjacent surrounding structures
- Time present, if known.

Making a radiological differential diagnosis depends on this systematic approach.

Comparison with previous films

The availability of previous films for comparative purposes is an invaluable aid to radiographic interpretation. The presence, extent and features of lesions can be compared to ascertain the speed of development and growth, or the degree of healing.

Note: Care must be taken that views used for comparison have been taken with a comparable technique **and** are of comparable density.

Conclusion

Successful interpretation of radiographs, no matter what the quality, relies ultimately on observers understanding the radiographic image, being able to recognize the range of normal appearances as well as knowing the salient features of relevant pathological conditions.

The following chapters are designed to emphasize these requirements and to reinforce the basic approach to interpretation outlined earlier.

18 Dental caries and the assessment of restorations

Introduction

Dental caries is usually classified by the area or site of the tooth that is affected. A common classification includes:

- Pit or fissure caries
  — Occlusal
  — Buccal or lingual pit
- Smooth surface caries
  — Approximal
  — Buccal or lingual surfaces
  — Root
- Recurrent caries.

The methods of diagnosing at these different sites include:

- Thorough, careful clinical examination, using:
  — Direct vision of clean, dry teeth
  — Gentle probing
  — Transillumination
- Radiographic examination, using:
  — Bitewings in adults and children
  — Paralleling technique periapicals in adults.

The first half of this chapter concentrates on the diagnosis of caries in posterior teeth from bitewing radiographs. The second half summarizes the important features to observe when assessing restorations and outlines a systematic approach to interpreting bitewing radiographs.

Carious lesions are detectable radiographically only when there has been enough demineralization to allow the lesion to be differentiated from normal enamel and dentine. The importance of utilizing optimum viewing conditions, as

described in Chapter 17, cannot be overemphasized when looking for these early subtle changes in radiodensity. Magnification is of particular importance, as shown in Figure 18.1.

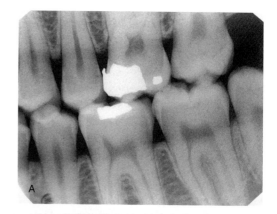

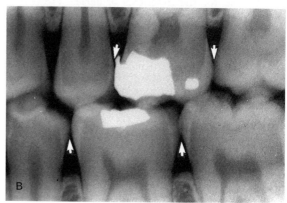

Fig. 18.1 The effect of magnification. **A** Bitewing radiograph showing almost invisible very early approximal lesions in the molar and premolar teeth. **B** Magnified central portion of the same bitewing showing the approximal lesions (arrowed) more clearly.

Radiographic appearance of caries

As carious lesions enlarge, they appear as different shaped areas of radiolucency in the crowns or necks of the teeth. These shapes are fairly characteristic and vary according to the *site* and *size* of the lesion. They are illustrated diagrammatically in Figure 18.2 and examples are shown in Figure 18.3.

Important points to note

• Radiographs are an invaluable AID to the diagnosis of caries and the assessment of restorations — a clinical examination alone will not suffice. However, over-reliance on radiographic information should be avoided.

• Radiographs, particularly bitewings, are also used to assess the progression of carious lesions. In the UK, the 1998 *Selection Criteria in Dental Radiography* booklet recommends that the frequency of these follow-up bitewings be linked to the *caries risk* of the patient. For high-caries-risk adult patients 6-monthly intervals are recommended, for medium-caries-risk patients 12-monthly intervals and for low-caries-risk patients 2-yearly intervals. Similar intervals are recommended for children with the exception of children considered at low caries risk, who should be radiographed at 12- to 18-monthly intervals in the primary dentition (see Ch. 6).

• Dental panoramic tomographs are not recommended for the diagnosis of caries. However, they may demonstrate occlusal caries, particularly in molars, better than bitewings. This may be because the carious lesion lies in the middle of the tomographic slice and is *in focus*, while the sound buccal and lingual surfaces of the tooth are blurred out and thus do not obscure the image.

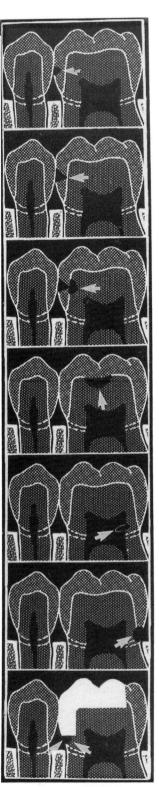

Approximal caries confined to enamel

Approximal caries extending to EDJ

Approximal caries extending into dentine

Occlusal caries extending into dentine. No obvious enamel shadow

Buccal/lingual caries

Root caries

Recurrent caries

Fig. 18.2 Diagrams illustrating the radiographic appearances and shapes of various carious lesions. EDJ, enamel–dentine junction.

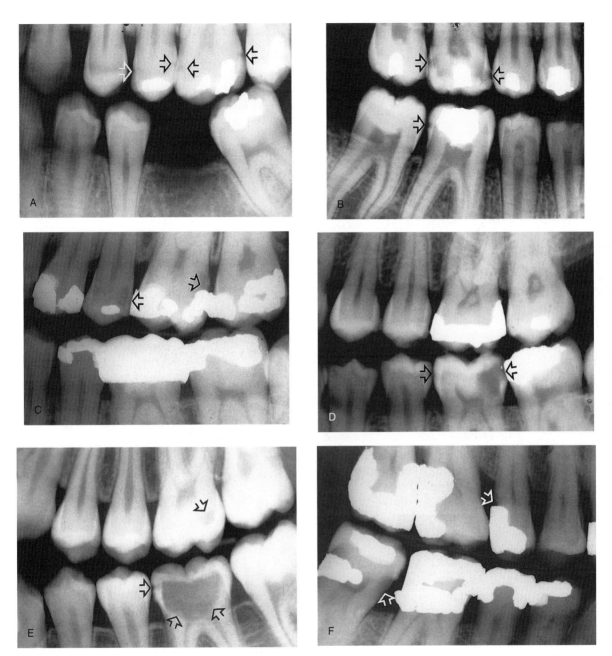

Fig. 18.3 Bitewing radiographs showing examples of typical carious lesions (arrowed). **A** Small approximal lesions $\underline{/56}$. **B** Large approximal lesions with extensive dentine involvement $\underline{6/}$ and a small lesion $\overline{6/}$. **C** Approximal lesion extending into dentine $\underline{/5}$ and recurrent caries $\underline{/6}$. **D** Small and extensive approximal lesions $\overline{/6}$. **E** Small occlusal lesion $\underline{/6}$ and extensive occlusal lesion $\overline{/6}$, apart from the small approximal enamel lesion, the enamel cap appears intact. **F** Root caries $\overline{7/}$ and recurrent caries $\underline{5/}$.

Radiographic appearance of other important shadows

Unfortunately, radiographic interpretation of dental caries is not always straightforward. It is often complicated by two additional radiographic shadows:

- Radiolucent cervical *burn-out* or *translucency*
- The radiopaque zone beneath amalgam restorations.

Radiolucent cervical burn-out

This radiolucent shadow is often evident at the neck of the teeth, as illustrated in Figure 18.4. It is an artefactual phenomenon created by the anatomy of the teeth and the variable penetration of the X-ray beam.

Cervical *burn-out* can be explained by considering **all** the different parts of the tooth and supporting bone tissues that the same X-ray beam has to penetrate:

- In the crown — the dense enamel cap and dentine
- In the neck — only dentine
- In the root — dentine and the buccal and lingual plates of alveolar bone (see Fig. 18.5).

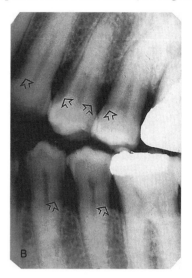

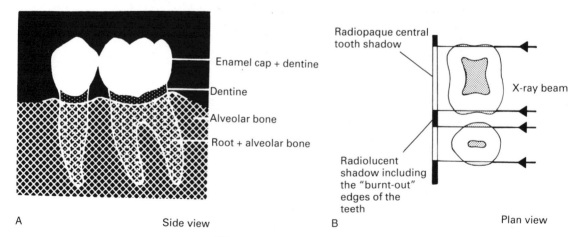

Fig. 18.4A Diagram illustrating the radiographic appearance of cervical *burn-out*. **B** Vertical bitewing radiograph showing extensive cervical burn-out, affecting particularly the premolars (arrowed).

Fig. 18.5A Diagrammatic representation of √5̅6̅ from the side showing the three-dimensional structures involved in the formation of the radiographic image. Note that in the cervical region there is less tissue present. **B** Plan view at the level of the necks of the teeth. Through the centre of the teeth there is a large mass of dentine to absorb the X-ray beam, while at the edges there is only a small amount. The edges of the necks of the teeth are therefore not dense enough to stop the X-ray beam, so their normally opaque shadows do not appear on the final radiograph.

Thus, at the edges of the teeth in the cervical region, there is **less** tissue for the X-ray beam to pass through. Less attenuation therefore takes place and virtually no opaque shadow is cast of this area on the radiograph. It therefore appears radiolucent, as if some cervical tooth tissue does not exist or that it has been apparently *burnt-out*.

Cervical *burn-out* is of diagnostic importance because of its similarity to the radiolucent shadows of cervical and recurrent caries. However, *burn-out* can usually be distinguished by the following characteristic features:

- It is located at the neck of the teeth, demarcated above by the enamel cap or restoration and below by the alveolar bone level
- It is triangular in shape, gradually becoming less apparent towards the centre of the tooth
- Usually all the teeth on the radiograph are affected, especially the smaller premolars.

In contrast, *root* and *recurrent carious lesions*, although they also often affect the cervical region, have no apparent upper and lower demarcating borders. These lesions are saucer-shaped and tend to be localized, as shown in Figure 18.2. If in doubt, the diagnosis should be confirmed clinically by direct vision and gentle probing having cleaned and dried the area.

Important points to note

- *Burn-out* is more obvious when the exposure factors are increased, as required ideally for detecting approximal caries.
- It is also more apparent by the perceptual problem of *contrast* if the tooth contains a metallic restoration, which may make the zone above the cervical shadow completely radiopaque (see Fig. 18.6 and Ch. 1, Fig. 1.16). As this area is also the main site for recurrent caries, diagnosis is further complicated.

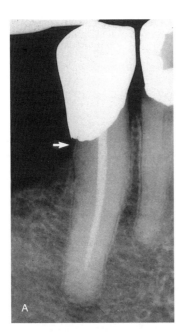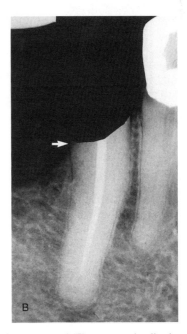

Fig. 18.6 The visual perceptual problem of contrast — **A** The zone at the distal cervical margin (arrowed), directly beneath the white metallic restoration shadow, appears radiolucent in the $\overline{5/}$. **B** The same image but with the white restoration blacked out. The zone beneath the restoration (arrowed) now appears less radiolucent.

Radiopaque zone beneath amalgam restorations

Following carious attack, posterior teeth are still most commonly restored using dental amalgam. An *amalgam* is defined as an alloy of mercury with another metal or metals. In dental amalgam, mercury is mixed with an alloy powder. The alloy powders available principally contain silver, tin and copper with small amounts of zinc. It has been shown that, with time, tin and zinc ions are released into the underlying demineralized (but not necessarily infected) dentine producing a radiopaque zone within the dentine which follows the S-shape curve of the underlying tubules (see Fig. 18.7). The radiopacity of this zone may make the normal dentine on either side appear more radiolucent by contrast. This somewhat more radiolucent normal dentine may simulate the radiolucent shadows of caries and lead to difficulties in diagnosis.

In addition, the pulp may also respond to both the carious attack and subsequent restorative treatment by laying down *reparative secondary dentine* which reduces the size of the pulp chamber.

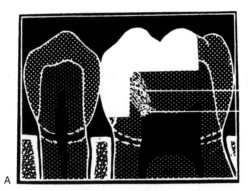

Radiopaque zone owing to Sn and Zn ions

Reparative dentine

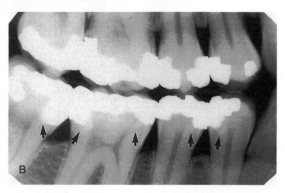

Fig. 18.7A Diagram illustrating the S-shaped radiopaque zone caused by tin and zinc ions released into the underlying demineralized dentine beneath an amalgam restoration and the appearance of reparative dentine.
B Bitewing radiograph showing the S-shaped radiopaque shadows (arrowed) in the heavily restored lower teeth.

Limitations of radiographic diagnosis of caries

In addition to the problems of diagnosis caused by the radiolucent and radiopaque shadows mentioned earlier, further limitations are imposed by the radiographic image. The main problems include:

- Carious lesions are usually larger clinically than they appear radiographically and very early lesions are not evident at all.
- Technique variations in film and X-ray beam positions can affect considerably the image of the carious lesion — varying the horizontal tubehead angulation can make a lesion confined to enamel appear to have progressed into dentine (see Fig. 18.8) — hence the need for accurate, reproducible techniques as described in Chapter 9.
- Exposure factors can have a marked effect on the overall radiographic contrast (see Fig. 18.9)

and thus affect the appearance or size of carious lesions on the radiograph.

- Superimposition and a two-dimensional image mean that the following features cannot always be determined:
  — The exact site of a carious lesion, e.g. buccal or lingual
  — The bucco-lingual extent of a lesion
  — The distance between the carious lesion and the pulp horns. These two shadows can appear to be close together or even in contact but they may not be in the same plane
  — The presence of an enamel lesion — the density of the overlying enamel may obscure the zone of decalcification
  — The presence of recurrent caries — existing restorations may completely overlie the carious lesion (see Fig. 18.10).

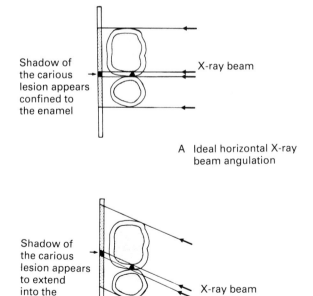

Shadow of the carious lesion appears confined to the enamel

X-ray beam

A Ideal horizontal X-ray beam angulation

Shadow of the carious lesion appears to extend into the dentine

X-ray beam

B Incorrect horizontal X-ray beam angulation

Fig. 18.8 Diagrams showing how the appearance and extent of a carious lesion confined to enamel alter with different horizontal X-ray beam angulations.

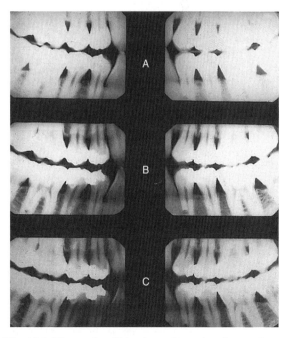

Fig. 18.9 Three pairs of bitewing radiographs taken on the same patient but with varying exposure factors.
A Considerably reduced exposure, **B** Slightly reduced exposure and **C** Slightly increased exposure. Note the varying contrast between enamel, dentine and the pulp.

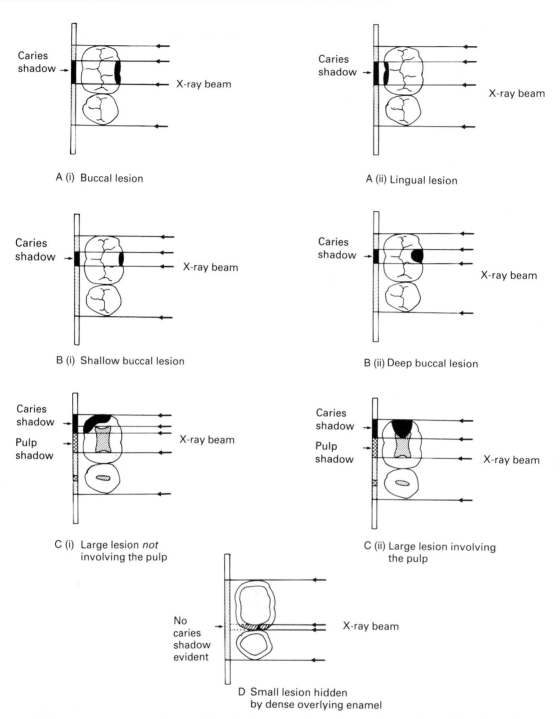

Fig. 18.10A Diagrams showing differently positioned lesions (i) buccal and (ii) lingual, producing similar radiographic shadows. **B** Diagrams showing different sized buccal lesions (i) shallow and (ii) deep, producing similar radiographic shadows. **C** Diagrams showing (i) a large approximal lesion superimposed over, but not involving the pulp and (ii) a large approximal lesion involving the pulp, both producing similar radiographic shadows. **D** Diagram showing how a small lesion may not be evident radiographically if dense radiopaque enamel shadows are superimposed.

Radiographic assessment of restorations

Critical assessment of the restoration

The important features to note include:

- The type and radiodensity of the restorative material, e.g.
  — amalgam
  — cast metal
  — tooth-coloured materials such as composite or glass ionomer
- Overcontouring
- Overhanging ledges
- Undercontouring
- Negative or reverse ledges
- Presence of contact points
- Adaptation of the restorative material to the base of the cavity

- Marginal fit of cast restorations
- Presence or absence of a lining material
- Radiodensity of the lining material.

Assessment of the underlying tooth

The important features to note include:

- Recurrent caries
- Residual caries
- Radiopaque shadow of released tin and zinc ions
- Size of the pulp chamber
- Internal resorption
- Presence of root-filling material in the pulp chamber
- Presence and position of pins or posts.

Examples showing several of these features are shown in Figure 18.11.

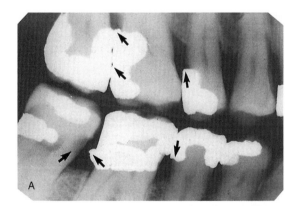
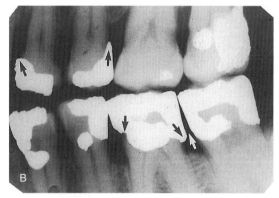
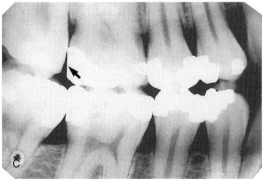
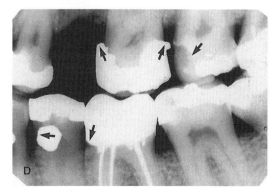

Fig. 18.11 Bitewing radiographs showing examples of heavily restored teeth. The major areas of concern — overhanging ledges, poor contour, defective contact points and recurrent caries — are arrowed.

Limitations of the radiographic image

Once again, the radiographic image provides only limited information when assessing restorations. The main problems include:

- Technique variations in X-ray tubehead position may cause recurrent carious lesions to be obscured (see Fig. 18.12)
- Cervical *burn-out* shadows tend to be more obvious when their upper borders are demarcated by dense white restorations because of the increased contrast differences (see Fig. 18.6)

- Superimposition and a two-dimensional image mean that:
  — Only part of a restoration can be assessed radiographically
  — A dense radiopaque restoration may totally obscure a carious lesion in another part of the tooth
  — Recurrent caries at the base of an interproximal box may not be detected (see Fig. 18.13).

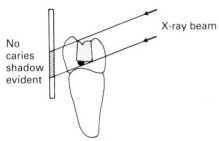

A Incorrect vertical X-ray beam angulation

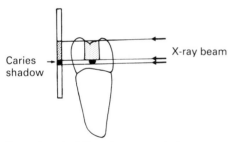

B Ideal vertical X-ray beam angulation

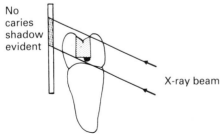

C Incorrect vertical X-ray beam angulation

Fig. 18.12 Diagrams illustrating the effect of incorrect vertical X-ray beam angulation in diagnosing recurrent lesions at the base of a restoration box.

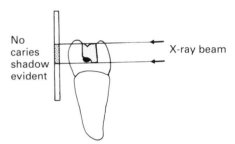

A (i) Lesion beneath the restoration

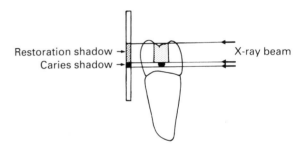

A (ii) Lesion hidden by the restoration

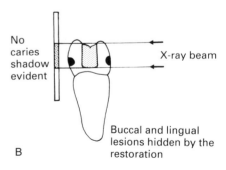

B

Fig. 18.13A Diagrams illustrating the difficulty of assessing caries beneath a restoration. **B** Diagram showing the difficulty of assessing buccal and lingual lesions in restored teeth.

Suggested guidelines for interpreting bitewing radiographs

Overall critical assessment

A typical series of questions that should be asked about the quality of a bitewing radiograph include:

Technique

- Are all the required teeth shown?
- Are the crowns of upper and lower teeth shown?
- Is the occlusal plane horizontal?
- Are the contact areas overlapped?
- Has there been any *coning off* or *cone cutting*?
- Are the buccal and lingual cusps overlapped?
- Is it geometrically comparable to previous films?

Exposure factors

- Is the image too dark — and so possibly overexposed?
- Is the image too light — and so possibly underexposed?
- Is the exposure sufficient to allow the enamel – dentine junction to be seen?
- What effect do the exposure factors have on the structures shown?
- How noticeable is the cervical *burn-out*?

Processing

- Is the radiograph correctly processed?
- Is it overdeveloped?
- Is it underdeveloped?
- Is it correctly fixed?
- Has it been adequately washed?

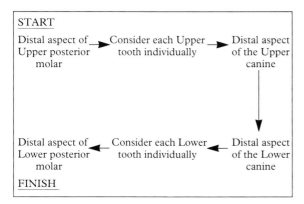

Fig. 18.14 Suggested sequence for examining a right bitewing radiograph.

Systematic viewing

Suggested systematic approaches to viewing bitewing radiographs are shown in Figures 18.14 and 18.15.

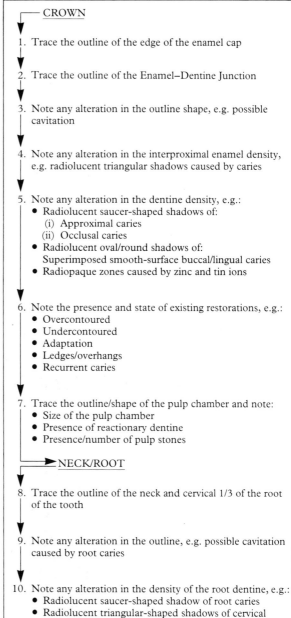

Fig. 18.15 Suggested sequence for examining each individual tooth.

19 The periapical tissues

Introduction

This chapter explains how to interpret the radiographic appearances of the periapical tissues by illustrating the various normal appearances, and describing in detail the typical changes associated with apical infection and inflammation following pulpal necrosis. To help explain the different radiographic appearances, they are correlated with the various underlying pathological processes. In addition, there is a summary of the other, sometimes sinister, lesions that can affect the periapical tissues and may simulate simple inflammatory changes.

Normal radiographic appearances

A reminder of the complex three-dimensional anatomy of the hard tissues surrounding the teeth in the maxilla and mandible, which contribute to the two-dimensional periapical radiographic image, is given in Figure 19.1.

The appearances of normal, healthy, periapical tissues vary from one patient to another, from one area of the mouth to another and at different stages in the development of the dentition. These different normal appearances are described below.

The periapical tissues of permanent teeth
(Fig. 19.2)

The three most important features to observe are:

- The radiolucent line that represents the periodontal ligament space and forms a thin continuous black line around the root outline

- The radiopaque line that represents the lamina dura of the bony socket and forms a thin, continuous, white line adjacent to the black line
- The trabecular pattern and density of the surrounding bone:
  — In the mandible, the trabeculae tend to be relatively thick and close together, and are often aligned horizontally
  — In the maxilla, the trabeculae tend to be finer, and more widely spaced. There is no predominant alignment pattern.

These features hold the key to the interpretation of periapical radiographs, since changes in their thickness, continuity and radiodensity reflect the presence of any underlying disease, as described later.

Important points to note

- There is considerable variation in the definition and pattern of these features from one patient to another and from one area of the jaws to another, owing to variation in the density, shape and thickness of the surrounding bone.
- The limitations imposed by contrast, resolution and superimposition can make radiographic identification of these features particularly difficult, hence the need for ideal viewing conditions.

The periapical tissues of deciduous teeth
(Fig. 19.3)

The important features of normality (thin lamina dura and periodontal ligament shadows) are the

197

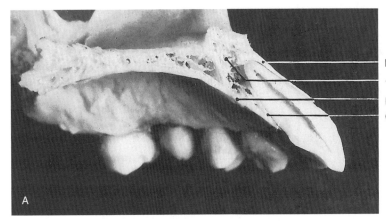

Buccal cortical plate of compact bone

Trabecular or cancellous bone
Palatal cortical plate of compact bone
Cortical bone of the socket

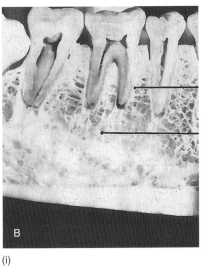

Cortical bone
of the
socket

Trabecular or
cancellous
bone

(i)

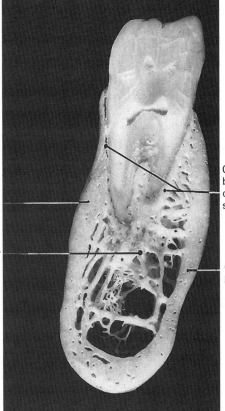

Cortical
bone
of the
socket

Lingual
cortical
plate

Buccal
cortical
plate

Trabecular or
cancellous
bone

(ii)

Fig. 19.1A Sagittal section through the maxilla and
central incisor showing the hard tissue anatomy. **B (i)**
Sagittal and **(ii)** coronal sections through the mandible
in the molar region showing the hard tissue anatomy.

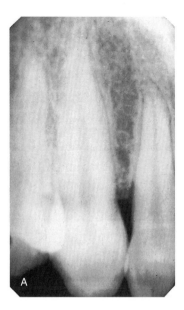

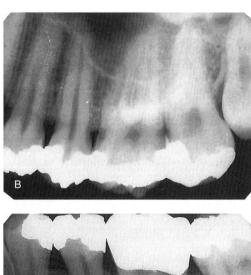

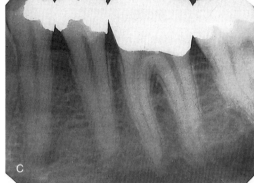

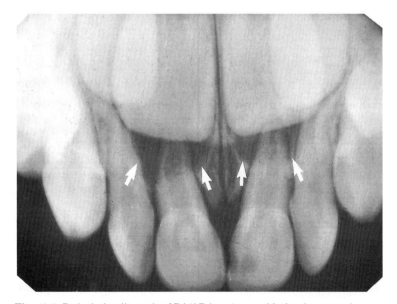

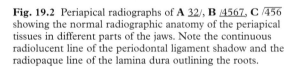

Fig. 19.2 Periapical radiographs of **A** <u>32</u>/, **B** /<u>4567</u>, **C** /456 showing the normal radiographic anatomy of the periapical tissues in different parts of the jaws. Note the continuous radiolucent line of the periodontal ligament shadow and the radiopaque line of the lamina dura outlining the roots.

Fig. 19.3 Periapical radiograph of <u>BA/AB</u> in a 4-year-old, showing normal periapical tissues. Note the confusing shadows created by the radiopaque crowns and radiolucent crypts (arrowed) of the developing permanent incisors.

same as for permanent teeth, but can be complicated by:

- The presence of an underlying permanent tooth and its crypt, the shadows of which may overlie the deciduous tooth apex
- Resorption of the deciduous tooth root during the normal exfoliation process.

The periapical tissues of developing teeth (Fig. 19.4)

The important features of normal apical tissues where the root is partially formed and the radicular papilla still exists include:

- A circumscribed area of radiolucency at the apex
- The radiopaque line of the lamina dura is intact around the papilla
- The developing root is funnel-shaped

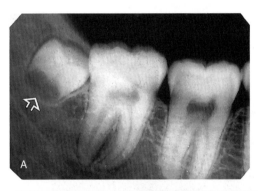

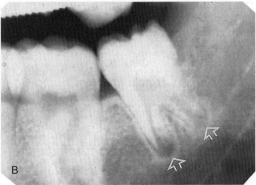

Fig. 19.4 Periapical radiographs showing the normal periapical tissues of developing teeth. **A** 8̄7̄, **B** /7. Note the circumscribed areas of radiolucency of the radicular papillae (arrowed) and the funnel-shaped roots.

- Only after root development is complete does the thin continuous radiolucent line become evident.

The effects of normal superimposed shadows

Normal anatomical shadows superimposed on the apical tissues can be either *radiolucent* or *radiopaque*, depending on the structure involved.

Radiolucent shadows

Examples include:

- The maxillary antra
- The nasopalatine foramen
- The mental foramina.

Such cavities in the alveolar bone decrease the total amount of bone that would normally contribute to the final radiographic image, with the following effects:

- The radiolucent line of the periodontal ligament may appear MORE radiolucent or widened, but will still be continuous and well demarcated
- The radiopaque line of the lamina dura may appear LESS obvious and may not be visible
- There will be an area of radiolucency in the alveolar bone at the tooth apex (see Figs 19.5 and 19.6).

Important points to note

- The fact that the radiopaque lamina dura shadow may not be visible does not mean that the bony socket margin is not present clinically. It only means that there is now not enough total bone in the path of the X-ray beam to produce a visible opaque shadow. Since the bony socket is in fact intact, it still defines the periodontal ligament space. Thus, the radiolucent line representing this space still appears continuous and well demarcated.
- Although confusing, this effect of normal anatomical radiolucent shadows on the apical tissues is very important to appreciate, so as not to mistake a normal area of radiolucency at the apex for a pathological lesion.

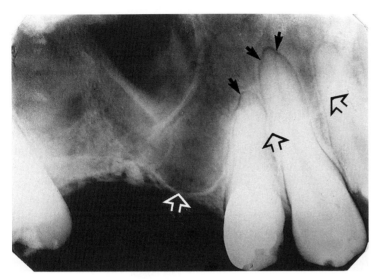

Fig. 19.5 Periapical of Q/ showing normal healthy apical tissues but with the radiolucent shadow of the antrum superimposed (the antral floor is indicated by the open arrows). As a result the radiolucent line of the periodontal ligament appears widened and more obvious around the apices of the canine and premolar, but it is still well demarcated, while the radiopaque line of the lamina dura is almost invisible (solid arrows).

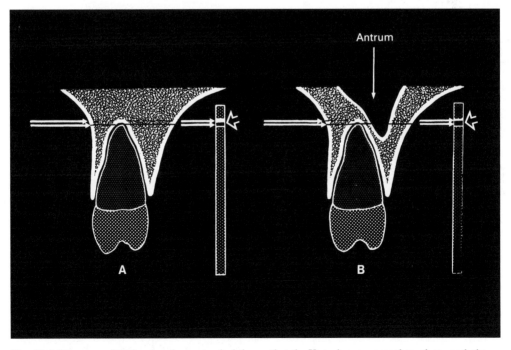

Fig. 19.6 Diagrams of 5/ showing the anatomical tissues that the X-ray beam passes through to reach the film. **A** Without a normal anatomical cavity superimposed. **B** With the antral cavity in the path of the X-ray beam. The different resultant radiopaque (white) and radiolucent (black) lines of the apical lamina dura and periodontal ligament are shown on the film (arrowed).

Radiopaque shadows

Examples include:

- The mylohyoid ridge
- The body of the zygoma
- Areas of sclerotic bone (so-called *dense bone islands*).

Such radiopacities complicate periapical interpretation by obscuring or obliterating the detailed shadows of the apical tissues, as shown in Figure 19.7.

Radiographic appearances of periapical inflammatory changes

Types of inflammatory changes

Following pulpal necrosis, either an acute or chronic inflammatory response is initiated in the apical tissues. The inflammatory response is identical to that set up elsewhere in the body from other toxic stimuli, and exhibits the same signs and symptoms.

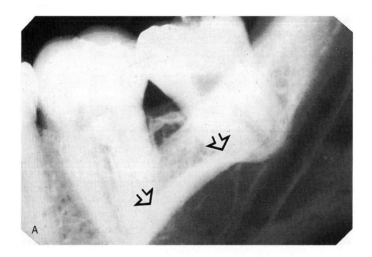

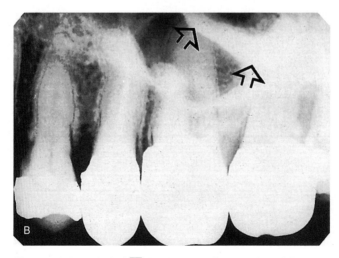

Fig. 19.7A Periapical of /78 showing the radiopaque line of the mylohyoid ridge (arrowed) superimposed over the apices. **B** Periapical of /4567 showing the radiopaque shadow of the zygomatic buttress (arrowed) overlying and obscuring the apical tissues of the molars.

Cardinal signs of acute inflammation

These include:

- Swelling — *tumor*
- Redness — *rubor*
- Heat — *calor*
- Pain — *dolor*
- Loss of function — *functio laesa*.

In the apical tissues, inflammatory exudate accumulates in the apical periodontal ligament space (*swelling*), setting up an **acute apical periodontitis**. The affected tooth becomes periostitic or tender to pressure (*pain*), and the patient avoids biting on the tooth (*loss of function*). *Heat* and *redness* are clinically undetectable. These signs are accompanied by destruction and resorption, often of the tooth root, and of the surrounding bone, as a **periapical abscess** develops, and radiographically a periapical radiolucent area becomes evident.

Hallmarks of chronic inflammation

These include the processes of *destruction* and *healing* which are going on simultaneously, as the body's defence systems respond to, and try to confine, the spread of the infection. In the apical tissues, a **periapical granuloma** forms at the apex and dense bone is laid down around the area of resorption. Radiographically, the apical radiolucent area becomes circumscribed and surrounded by dense sclerotic bone. Occasionally, under these conditions of chronic inflammation, the epithelial cell rests of Malassez are stimulated to proliferate and form an inflammatory **periapical radicular cyst** or there is an acute exacerbation producing another abscess (the so-called *phoenix abscess*).

The type and progress of the inflammatory response at the apex and the subsequent spread of apical infection is dependent on several factors relating to:

- The infecting organism including its virulence
- The body's defence systems.

The result is a wide spectrum of events ranging from a very rapidly spreading acute periapical abscess to a very slowly progressing chronic periapical granuloma or cyst. This variation in the underlying disease processes is mirrored radiographically, although it is often not possible to differentiate between an abscess, granuloma or cyst.

A summary of the different inflammatory effects and the resultant radiographic appearances is shown in Table 19.1. The effects are shown diagrammatically in Figure 19.8. Various examples are shown in Figures 19.9–19.12.

Table 19.1 Summary of the effects of different inflammatory processes on the periapical tissues and the resultant radiographic appearances

State of inflammation	Underlying inflammatory changes	Radiographic appearances
Initial acute inflammation	Inflammatory exudate accumulates in the apical periodontal ligament space — *acute apical periodontitis*	Widening of the radiolucent line of the periodontal ligament space OR No apparent changes evident
Initial spread of inflammation	Resorption and destruction of the apical bony socket — *periapical abscess*	Loss of the radiopaque line of the lamina dura at the apex
Further spread of inflammation	Further resorption and destruction of the apical alveolar bone	Area of bone loss at the tooth apex
Initial low-grade chronic inflammation	Minimal destruction of the apical bone The body's defence systems lay down dense bone in the apical region	No apparent bone destruction but dense sclerotic bone evident around the tooth apex (*sclerosing osteitis*)
Latter stages of chronic inflammation	Apical bone is resorbed and destroyed and dense bone is laid down around the area of resorption — *periapical granuloma* or *radicular cyst*	Circumscribed, well-defined radiolucent area of bone loss at the apex, surrounded by dense sclerotic bone

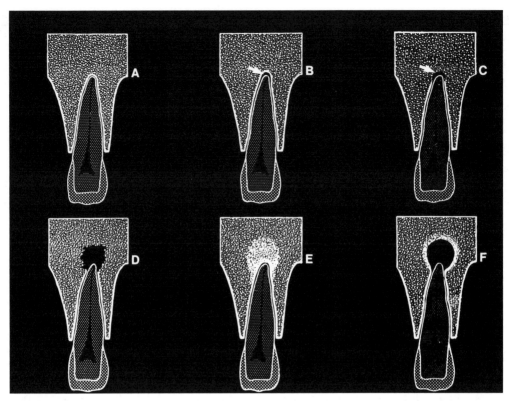

Fig. 19.8 Diagrams showing the various radiographic appearances of infection and inflammation in the apical tissues. **A** Normal. **B** Early apical change — widening of the radiolucent periodontal ligament space (*acute apical periodontitis*) (arrowed). **C** Early apical change — loss of the radiopaque lamina dura (*early periapical abscess*) (arrowed). **D** Extensive destructive acute inflammation — diffuse, ill-defined area of radiolucency at the apex (*periapical abscess*). **E** Low grade chronic inflammation — diffuse radiopaque area at the apex (*sclerosing osteitis*). **F** Longstanding chronic inflammation — well-defined area of radiolucency surrounded by dense sclerotic bone (*periapical granuloma or radicular cyst*).

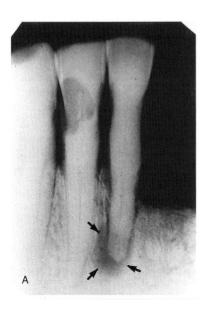

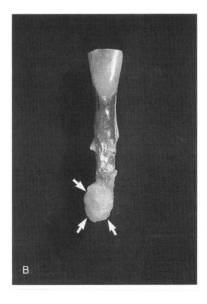

Fig. 19.9A Periapical showing a well-defined area of radiolucency at the apex of $\overline{7|}$ (arrowed). The surrounding bone is relatively dense and opaque suggesting a chronic periapical granuloma or radicular cyst. **B** The extracted $\overline{7|}$, showing the granuloma attached to the root apex (arrowed).

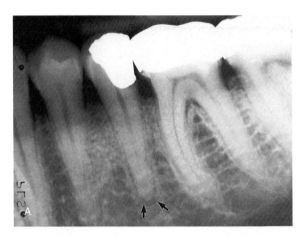
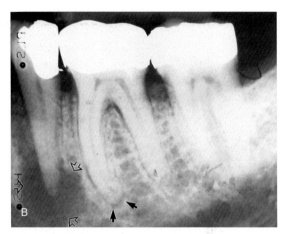

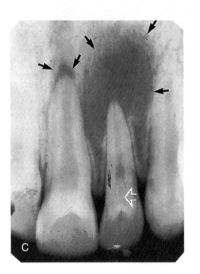
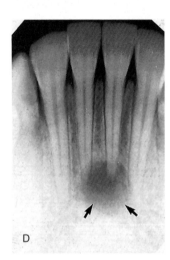

Fig. 19.10 Periapicals showing examples of inflammatory changes in the periapical tissues. **A** Early apical change on $\overline{5}$ showing widening of the periodontal ligament space and thinning of the lamina dura (*acute apical periodontitis*) (arrowed). **B** Same patient 6 months later — the area of bone destruction at the apex $\overline{5}$ has increased considerably (open arrows) and there is now early apical change associated with the mesial root $\overline{6}$ (solid arrows). **C** Large, diffuse area of bone destruction associated with $\underline{2}$ and a smaller area associated with $\underline{1}$ (black arrows) (*periapical abscess*). $\underline{2}$ shows evidence of a dens-in-dente (invaginated odontome) (open white arrow). **D** Reasonably well-defined area of bone destruction (arrowed) associated with $\overline{1}$ (*periapical abscess, granuloma or cyst*).

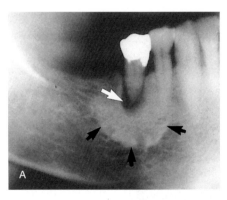
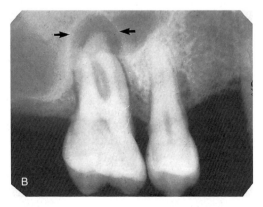

Fig. 19.11 Radiographic examples of other chronic inflammatory changes in the periapical tissues. **A** Long-standing low grade chronic infection associated with $\overline{5}$ resulting in a radiolucent periapical granuloma or radicular cyst (white arrow), surrounded by florid opaque sclerosing osteitis (black arrow). **B** Well-defined area of bone destruction associated with $\underline{6}$ which has resulted in remodelling of the antral floor, producing the so-called *antral halo* appearance (black arrow).

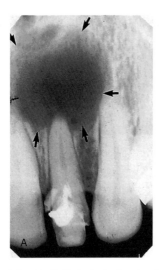 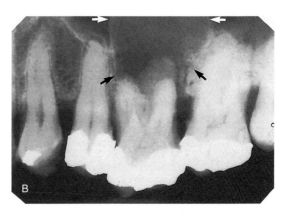

Fig. 19.12 Periapicals showing **A** Inflammatory radicular cyst (arrowed) associated with 2/. **B** Inflammatory radicular cyst (arrowed) associated with /6. The antrum has been displaced by the upper margin of the cyst which is not evident on this radiograph.

Treatment and radiographic follow-up

Conventional endodontic therapy which involves orthograde root canal debridement, to remove the source of the infection followed by obturation and sealing of the canals to prevent recontamination, is now used to treat initially most inflammatory periapical areas. The 1998 UK *Selection Criteria in Dental Radiography* booklet recommended at least one immediate postoperative radiograph to assess the success of the obturation and to act as a baseline for assessment of apical disease or healing. In addition, follow-up radiographs were recommended to be taken at 1 year and 4 years after completion of treatment (see Fig. 19.13). These films should ideally be taken using a similar technique and with the same exposure factors.

If endodontic therapy is clinically unsuccessful, subsequent treatment involves either:

- Surgical exploration, curettage of the infected area and/or enucleation of the cyst, apicectomy and retrograde rootfilling
- Extraction of the tooth.

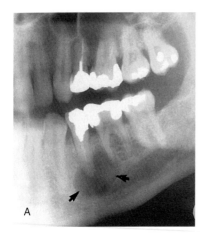 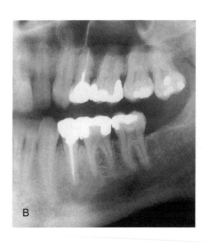

Fig. 19.13A Part of a dental panoramic tomograph showing a round, well-defined area of radiolucency — a likely radicular cyst (arrowed), associated with the poorly root-filled /5. **B** Same patient 6 months later following successful root filling at /5. Note the bony fill-in in the apical area.

Other important causes of periapical radiolucency

Many of the conditions illustrated in Chapter 22 can present occasionally in the apical region of the alveolar bone. Some can simulate the simple inflammatory changes described above including:

- Benign and malignant bone tumours including secondary metastatic deposits (see Fig. 19.14)
- Lymphoreticular tumours of bone
- Langerhans cell disease
- Fibro-cemento-osseous lesions.

Although it is uncommon, dental nurses should still be alert to the possibility that malignant lesions can present as apparently simple localized areas of infection. The signs of concern include:

- A vital tooth with minimal caries
- Spiking root resorption and an irregular radiolucent apical area with a ragged, poorly defined outline
- Tooth mobility in the absence of generalized periodontal disease
- Regional nerve anaesthesia
- Failure to respond to good endodontic therapy.

Suggested guidelines for interpreting periapical radiographs

Although somewhat repetitive, this methodical approach to radiographic interpretation is so important, and so often ignored, that it is described again.

Overall critical assessment

A typical series of questions that should be asked about the quality of a periapical radiograph include:

Technique

- Is the required tooth shown?
- Is the apical alveolar bone shown?
- Has the film been taken using the bisected angle or paralleling technique?
- How much distortion is present?
- Is the image foreshortened or elongated?
- Are the crowns overlapped?
- Has there been any *coning off* or *cone cutting?*

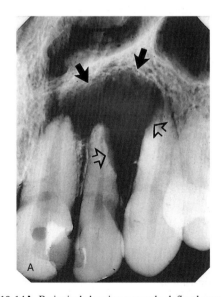

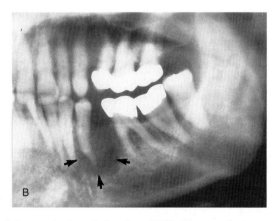

Fig. 19.14A Periapical showing a poorly defined area of radiolucency in the apical region of /123. Features of concern are the ragged bone margin (solid arrows) and the extensive resorption of /2 and /3 (open arrows). Initial treatment involved unsuccessful root treatment of /1. Biopsy revealed an osteosarcoma. **B** Part of a dental panoramic tomograph showing a large poorly defined area of radiolucency in /45 region (arrowed). Both premolars were caries-free and unrestored, but mobile. /5 was extracted and histopathology revealed a secondary metastatic malignant tumour from a breast primary.

Exposure factors

- Is the image too dark and so possibly overexposed?
- Is the image too light and so possibly underexposed?
- What effect do the exposure factors have on the appearance of the apical tissues?

Processing

- Is the radiograph correctly processed?
- Is it overdeveloped?
- Is it underdeveloped?
- Is it correctly fixed?
- Has it been adequately washed?

Systematic viewing

A systematic approach to viewing periapical radiographs is shown in Figure 19.15. This approach ensures that **all** areas of the film are observed and that the important features of the tooth apex are examined.

GENERAL OVERVIEW OF ENTIRE RADIOGRAPH
1. Note the chronological and development age of the patient
2. Note the position, outline and density of all the normal superimposed anatomical shadows including any developing teeth

EXAMINE EACH TOOTH ON THE RADIOGRAPH AND ASSESS

3. THE CROWN
   Note particularly:
   - The presence of caries
   - The state of existing restorations

4. THE ROOT(S)
   Note particularly:
   - The length of the root
   - The number(s)
   - The morphology
   - The size and shape of canals
   - The presence of:
     a. Pulp stones
     b. Root fillings
     c. Internal resorption
     d. External resorption
     e. Root fractures

5. THE APICAL TISSUES
   Note particularly:
   - The integrity, continuity and thickness of:
     a. The radiolucent line of the periodontal ligament space
     b. The radiopaque line of the lamina dura
   - Any associated radiolucent areas
   - Any associated radiopaque areas
   - The pattern of the trabecular bone

6. THE PERIODONTAL TISSUES
   Note particularly:
   - The width of the periodontal ligament
   - The level and quality of the crestal bone
   - Any vertical or horizontal bone loss
   - Any calculus deposits
   - Any furcation involvements

Fig. 19.15 A systematic sequence for viewing periapical radiographs.

20 The periodontal tissues and periodontal disease

Introduction

An overall assessment of the periodontal tissues is based on both the clinical examination and radiographic findings — the two investigations complement one another. Unfortunately, like many other indicators of periodontal disease, radiographs only provide retrospective evidence of the disease process. However, they can be used to assess the morphology of the affected teeth and the pattern and degree of alveolar bone loss that has taken place. *Bone loss* can be defined as *the difference between the present septal bone height and the assumed normal bone height for any particular patient*, taking age into account. In fact radiographs actually show the amount of alveolar bone *remaining* in relation to the length of the root. But this information is still important in the overall assessment of the severity of the disease, the prognosis of the teeth and for treatment planning.

Radiographs are therefore used to:

- Assess the extent of bone loss and furcation involvement
- Determine the presence of any secondary local causative factors
- Assist in treatment planning
- Evaluate treatment measures particularly following *guided tissue regeneration* (GTR).

The main radiographic projections used to show the periodontal tissues include:

- *Paralleling technique periapicals* (see Ch. 8)
- *Bitewings* — horizontal or vertical, normally for posterior teeth (see Ch. 9)

- *Dental panoramic tomographs*, where there is pocketing greater than 5 mm in depth (see Ch. 13)
- *Digital radiography* — including subtraction radiography and densitometric image analysis which may assist in showing and measuring subtle changes in fine alveolar and crestal bone pattern (see Ch. 16).

Once again, before any detailed interpretation is undertaken, the *quality* of the radiographs should be assessed in relation to:

- Technique
- Exposure factors — remembering that these should be reduced sufficiently to avoid *burn-out* of the interdental crestal bone, as shown in Figure 20.1
- Processing.

In the interpretation of the periodontal tissues, films of excellent quality are essential — perhaps more so than in other dental specialities — because of the fine detail that is required.

Radiographic features of healthy periodontium

A *healthy* periodontium can be regarded as *periodontal tissue exhibiting no evidence of disease*. Unfortunately, *health* cannot be ascertained from radiographs alone, clinical information is also required.

However, to be able to interpret radiographs successfully observers need to know the usual radiographic features of healthy tissues where there has been no bone loss. The only reliable

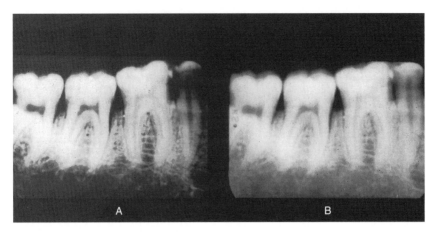

Fig. 20.1 Two periapical radiographs of the same patient, taken using the same technique but with different exposure factors. **A** Increased exposure. **B** Reduced exposure. Note the variation in the appearance of the interdental bone as a result of *burn-out*.

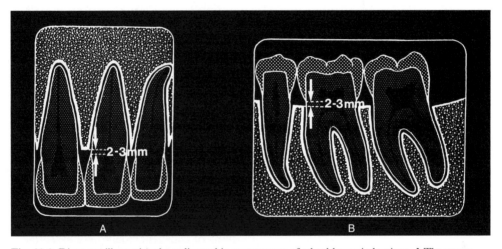

Fig. 20.2 Diagrams illustrating the radiographic appearances of a healthy periodontium. **A** The upper incisor region. **B** The lower molar region. The normal distance of 2–3 mm from the crestal margin to the cemento–enamel junction is indicated.

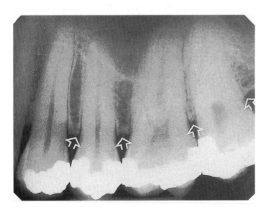

Fig. 20.3 Paralleling technique periapical radiograph of /4567 , (slightly reduced exposure) showing the radiographic features of a healthy periodontium (arrowed) before the onset of periodontitis.

radiographic feature is the relationship between the crestal bone margin and the cemento–enamel junction (CEJ). If this distance is within normal limits (2–3 mm) and there are no clinical signs of loss of attachment, then it can be said that there has been no periodontitis.

The usual radiographic features of *healthy* alveolar bone are shown in Figures 20.2 and 20.3 and include:

- Thin, smooth, evenly corticated margins to the interdental crestal bone in the posterior regions.
- Thin, even, pointed margins to the interdental crestal bone in the anterior regions.
  Cortication at the top of the crest is not always evident, owing mainly to the small amount of bone between the teeth anteriorly.
- The interdental crestal bone is continuous with the lamina dura of the adjacent teeth. The junction of the two forms a sharp angle.
- Thin even width to the mesial and distal periodontal ligament spaces.

Important points to note

- Although these are the usual features of a healthy periodontium, they are not always evident.
- Their absence from radiographs does not necessarily mean that periodontal disease is present
- Failure to see these features may be due to:
- — Technique error
- — Overexposure
- — Normal anatomical variation in alveolar bone shape and density.
- Following successful treatment, the periodontal tissues may appear healthy clinically, but radiographs may show evidence of earlier bone loss when the disease was active. Bone loss observed on radiographs is therefore not an indicator of the presence of inflammation.

Classification of periodontal disease

Various classifications of periodontal disease have been put forward over the years. The system favoured by the author is based on that found in *Proceedings of the 1st European Workshop in Periodontology* (eds N. Lang and T. Korning).

Inflammatory periodontal disease

Gingivitis

- Acute
  - — Caused by trauma
  - — Acute ulcerative gingivitis
  - — Acute herpetic gingivostomatitis
  - — Acute non-specific
- Chronic
  - — Hyperplastic
  - — Desquamative.

Periodontitis

- Acute
  - — Acute periodontal abscess
- Chronic periodontitis
  - — Early
  - — Moderate
  - — Severe
- Early onset periodontitis
  - — Pre-pubertal
  - — Juvenile
  - — Rapidly progressive.

Systemic or generalized conditions that can affect the periodontium

Including amongst others:

- Pregnancy
- Uncontrolled diabetes
- Drugs, e.g. Epanutin, nifedipine
- HIV
- Leukaemia
- Down's syndrome
- Langerhans cell disease (histiocytosis X)
- Papillon–Lefèvre syndrome
- Secondary metastases.

Radiographic features or periodontal disease and the assessment of bone loss and furcation involvement

Acute and chronic gingivitis

Radiographs provide no direct evidence of the soft tissue involvement in gingivitis. However, in severe cases of acute ulcerative gingivitis (AUG) where there has been extensive cratering of the interdental papilla, inflammatory destruction of the underlying crestal bone may be observed.

Periodontitis

Periodontitis is the name given to periodontal disease when *the superficial inflammation in the gingival tissues extends into the underlying alveolar bone and there has been loss of attachment.* The destruction of the bone can be either *localized*, affecting a few areas of the mouth, or *generalized* affecting all areas. The rate of this progression and subsequent bone destruction is usually slow and continues intermittently over many years or it may be rapid. The radiographic features of the different forms of periodontitis are similar; it is the distribution and the rate of bone destruction that varies.

Terminology

The terms used to describe the various appearances of bone destruction include:

- Horizontal bone loss
- Vertical bone loss
- Furcation involvements.

The terms *horizontal* and *vertical* have been used traditionally to describe the direction or pattern of bone loss using the line joining two adjacent teeth at their cemento-enamel junctions as a line of reference. The amount of bone loss is then assessed as mild, moderate or severe as shown diagrammatically in Figure 20.4. Severe vertical bone loss, extending from the alveolar crest and involving the tooth apex, in which necrosis of pulp tissue is also believed to be a contributory factor, is described as a *perio-endo lesion* (see Figs 20.4E and 20.6).

The term *furcation involvement* describes the radiographic appearance of bone loss in the furcation area of the roots which is evidence of advanced disease in this zone, as shown diagrammatically in Figure 20.5. Although central furcation involvements are seen more readily in mandibular molars, they can also be seen in maxillary molars despite the superimposed shadow of the overlying palatal root. In addition, early maxillary molar furcation involvement between the mesiobuccal or distobuccal roots and the palatal

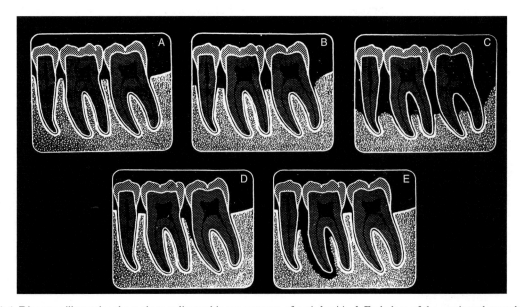

Fig. 20.4 Diagrams illustrating the various radiographic appearances of *periodontitis*. **A** Early loss of the corticated crestal bone, widening of the periodontal ligament and loss of the normally sharp angle between the crestal bone and the lamina dura. **B** Moderate horizontal bone loss. **C** Extensive generalized horizontal bone loss with furcation involvement. **D** Localized vertical bone loss affecting /7. **E** Extensive localized bone loss involving the apex of /6 — the so-called *perio-endo* lesion.

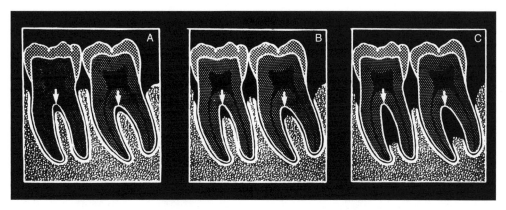

Fig. 20.5 Diagrams illustrating the radiographic appearances of varying degrees of furcation involvement in lower molars (arrowed). **A** Very early involvement showing widening of the furcation periodontal ligament shadow. **B** Moderate involvement. **C** Severe involvement.

root produces a characteristic triangular-shaped radiolucency at the edge of the tooth (see Figs 20.8C and 20.10A).

The typical radiographic features of three types of periodontitis, namely:

- Acute periodontitis — acute periodontal abscess
- Chronic periodontitis
- Early onset juvenile periodontitis
  are shown below:

Acute periodontitis — acute periodontal abscess

Occasionally, a patient may present with a local-ized acute exacerbation of underlying peri-odontal disease, usually originating in a deep soft tissue pocket which may have become occluded. The diagnosis of a periodontal abscess is made clinically where the signs of acute inflammation and infection are evident and not radiographi-cally, since the underlying radiographic bone changes may be indistinguishable from other forms of periodontal bone destruction, as shown in Figure 20.6.

Chronic periodontitis

This is the most common and important form of periodontal disease, affecting the majority of the dentate and partially dentate population. It is the main cause of loss of teeth in later adult life. The main pathological features of this disease are:

- Inflammation (usually a progression from chronic gingivitis)
- Destruction of periodontal ligament fibres
- Resorption of the alveolar bone
- Loss of epithelial attachment
- Formation of pockets around the teeth
- Gingival recession.

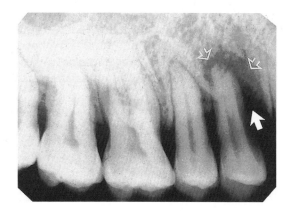

Fig. 20.6 Periapical radiograph showing an extensive area of bone loss (arrowed) associated with 4/ — a so-called *perio-endo* lesion. The patient had presented clinically with a periodontal abscess.

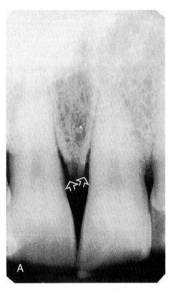 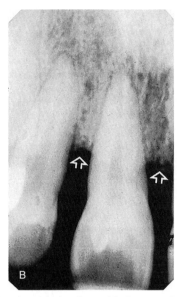

Fig. 20.7 Periapical radiographs showing the typical radiographic features of horizontal bone loss (arrowed) in periodontitis affecting maxillary incisors. **A** Moderate bone loss. **B** Severe bone loss.

It is the resorption of the alveolar bone that provides the main radiographic features of chronic periodontitis. These are illustrated in Figures 20.7–20.10 and include:

- Loss of the corticated interdental crestal margin, the bone edge becomes irregular or blunted
- Widening of the periodontal ligament space at the crestal margin
- Loss of the normally sharp angle between the crestal bone and the lamina dura — the bone angle becomes rounded and irregular
- Localized or generalized loss of the alveolar supporting bone
- Patterns of bone loss — *horizontal* and/or *vertical* — resulting in an even loss of bone or the formation of complex intra-bony defects
- Loss of bone in the furcation areas of multirooted teeth — this can vary from widening of the furcation periodontal ligament to large zones of bone destruction

- Widening of the interdental periodontal ligament spaces
- Associated complicating *secondary local factors* — although the primary cause of periodontal disease is bacterial plaque, many complicating secondary local factors may also be involved. Some of these factors can be detected on radiographs (see Fig. 20.11) and include:
  — Calculus deposits
  — Carious cavities
  — Overhanging filling ledges
  — Poor restoration margins
  — Lack of contact points
  — Poor restoration contour, including pontic design
  — Perforations by pins or posts
  — Endodontic status in relation to perio-endo lesions
  — Overerupted opposing teeth
  — Tilted teeth
  — Root approximation
  — Gingivally fitting partial dentures.

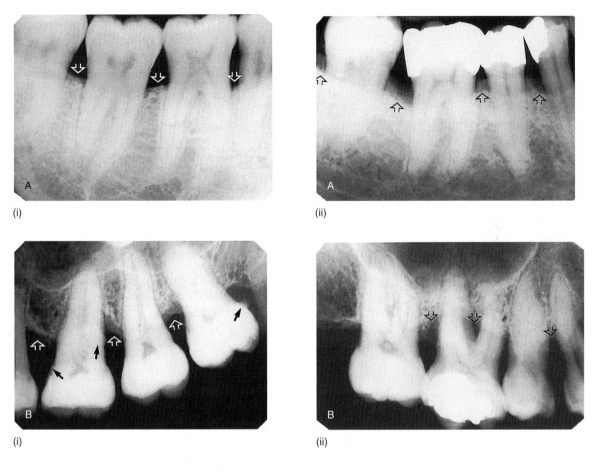

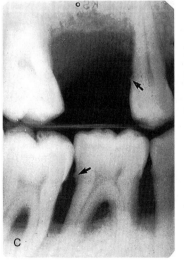

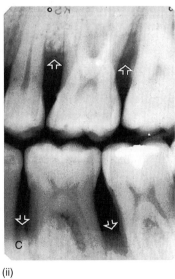

Fig. 20.8 Radiographs showing the typical radiographic features of horizontal bone loss in chronic periodontitis affecting posterior teeth. **A** (i) Early or mild and (ii) moderate bone loss (arrowed) affecting mandibular molars. **B** (i) Moderate and (ii) severe bone loss (open arrows) affecting maxillary molars. The black arrows indicate calculus deposits. **C** (i) and (ii) Vertical bitewings showing severe generalized bone loss (open arrows). The black arrows again indicate calculus deposits.

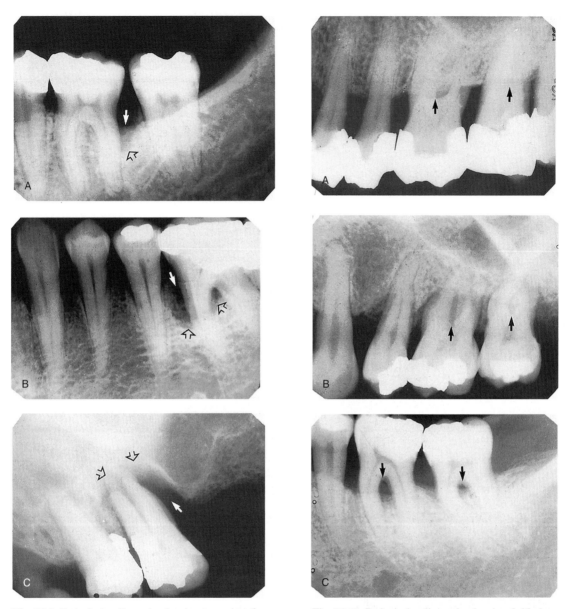

Fig. 20.9 Periapical radiographs showing examples of vertical bone loss in chronic periodontitis — **A** Mild/ moderate. **B** Moderate. **C** Severe localized defects (arrowed).

Fig. 20.10 Periapical radiographs showing **A** Moderate furcation involvement (black arrows) in maxillary molars. Note the characteristic mesial and distal cervical triangular radiolucent shadows indicating furcation involvement between the mesio-buccal and palatal roots and the distobuccal and palatal roots. **B** Severe degrees of furcation bone loss (arrowed) in maxillary molars. **C** Moderate and severe degrees of furcation bone loss (arrowed) in mandibular molars.

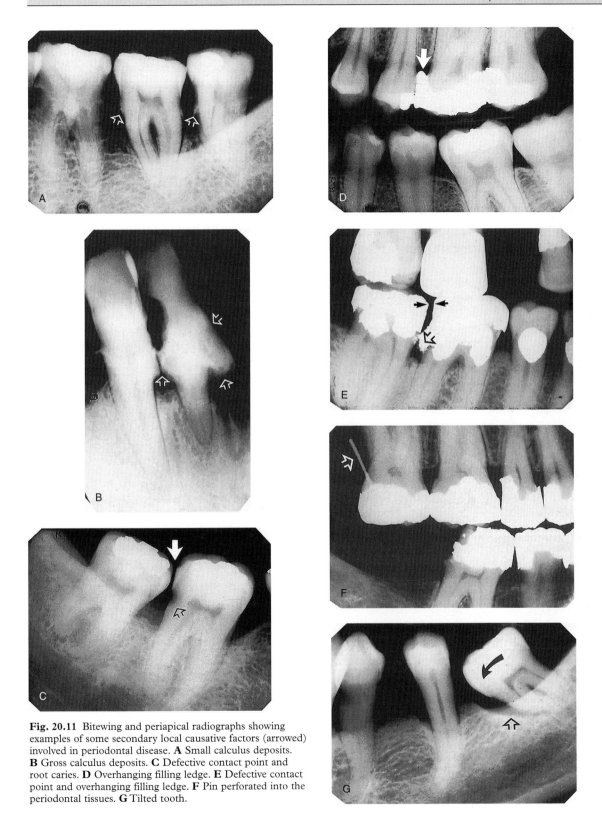

Fig. 20.11 Bitewing and periapical radiographs showing examples of some secondary local causative factors (arrowed) involved in periodontal disease. **A** Small calculus deposits. **B** Gross calculus deposits. **C** Defective contact point and root caries. **D** Overhanging filling ledge. **E** Defective contact point and overhanging filling ledge. **F** Pin perforated into the periodontal tissues. **G** Tilted tooth.

Early onset juvenile periodontitis

This localized severe form of periodontal disease develops in adolescence. An example is shown in Figure 20.12. Radiographic features include:

- Severe vertical bone defects affecting the first molars and/or incisors
- Arch or saucer-shaped defects
- Sometimes the bone loss is more generalized
- Migration of the incisors with diastema formation
- Rapid rate of bone loss.

Evaluation of treatment measures

Traditional treatment of periodontal disease involves improving oral hygiene, scaling, polishing and root planing of affected teeth surfaces and the removal of any other secondary local factors in an attempt to slow down or arrest the disease process. In recent years, there has been an attempt to achieve the ultimate treatment aim of regeneration of lost tissue by the development of the procedure called *guided tissue regeneration*. This favours regeneration of the attachment complex to denuded root surfaces by allowing selective regrowth of periodontal ligament cells while excluding the gingival tissues from reaching contact with the root during wound healing. This is achieved by surgically interposing a barrier membrane between the gingiva and the root surface.

The success or otherwise of these treatment measures can be assessed by a combination of clinical examination, including probing and

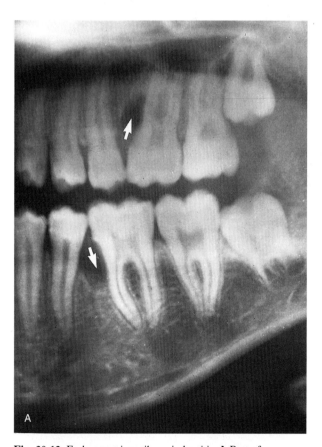

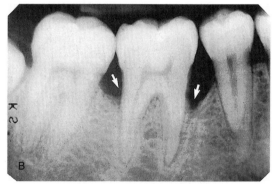

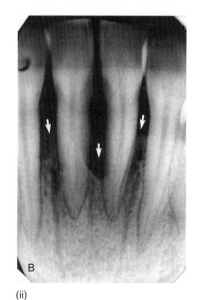

Fig. 20.12 Early onset juvenile periodontitis. **A** Part of a dental panoramic tomograph showing the typical bone defects affecting the first molars (arrowed). **B** Periapicals showing other typical bone defects (i) right mandibular molar and (ii) mandibular central incisors.

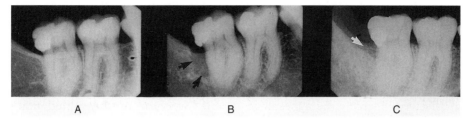

Fig. 20.13 Periapicals showing evaluation of treatment. **A** Initial film. **B** 9 years later showing overhanging filling margin and distal bony defect on $\overline{7|}$ (arrowed). **C** Follow-up film 3 years later following guided tissue regeneration showing the reduced defect (arrowed) and the bone in-fill. (Kindly supplied by Dr A. Sidi.)

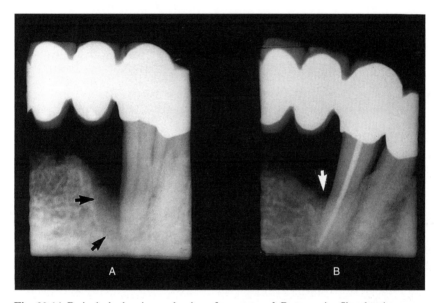

Fig. 20.14 Periapicals showing evaluation of treatment. **A** Preoperative film showing a perio-endo lesion affecting $/\overline{3}$ with severe bony defect on the mesial aspect of the root (arrowed). **B** Follow-up film 2 years later following successful endodontic therapy and guided tissue regeneration. Note the reduced bony defect (arrowed). (Kindly supplied by Dr A. Sidi.)

attachment loss measurements, and periodic radiographic investigation, as shown in Figures 20.13 and 20.14. **Note**: To provide useful information sequential radiographs ideally should be comparable in both technique and exposure factors.

Limitations of radiographic diagnosis

Radiographic evaluation of the periodontal tissues is somewhat limited. The main limitations include:

- Superimposition and a two-dimensional image bringing about the following problems:

— It is difficult to differentiate between the buccal and lingual crestal bone levels
— Only part of a complex bony defect is shown
— One wall of a bone defect may obscure the rest of the defect
— Dense tooth or restoration shadows may obscure buccal or lingual bone defects, and buccal or lingual calculus deposits
— Bone resorption in the furcation area may be obscured by an overlying root or bone shadow.

- Information is provided only on the hard tissues of the periodontium, since the soft tissue gingival defects are not normally detectable.

• Bone loss is detectable only when sufficient calcified tissue has been resorbed to alter the attenuation of the X-ray beam. As a result, the histological front of the disease process cannot be determined by the radiographic appearance.

• Technique variations in film and X-ray beam positions can affect considerably the appearance of the periodontal tissues; hence the need for accurate, reproducible techniques as described in Chapter 9.

• Exposure factors can have a marked effect on the apparent crestal bone height — overexposure causing *burn-out* as shown earlier in Figure 20.1.

• Complete reliance cannot be placed on the inherently inferior images of dental panoramic tomographs although they do provide a reasonable overview of the periodontal status (see Fig. 20.15 and Ch. 13).

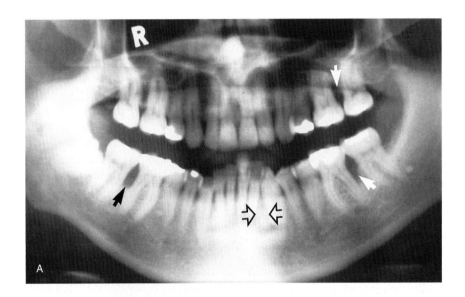

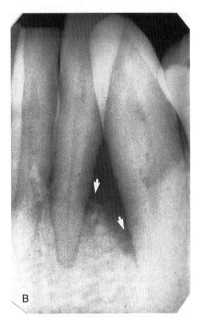

Fig. 20.15 A Dental panoramic tomograph showing bony defects in the molar regions (arrowed) but no evidence of a similar defect in the /23 region (open arrows) owing to superimposition of the radiopaque artefactual shadow of the cervical vertebrae. **B** Periapical of /23 region taken at the same time showing the severe bony defect (arrowed) that was actually present.

21 Implant assessment

Introduction

The restoration of edentulous and partially dentate jaws using a variety of implant-retained prostheses has become a relatively common clinical procedure in recent years. The implants are usually made of titanium and are described as either:

- Endosteal — placed **in** the bone. These are manufactured in a variety of shapes — screw, smooth-sided or plate-form, and essentially replace the roots of one or more teeth
- Subperiosteal — placed **on** the bone, under the periosteum and secured in place with screws.

This chapter concentrates on endosteal dental implants which are more commonly used, particularly since P. I. Brånemark's clinical research on the concept of *osseointegration* which he defined as *a direct connection between living bone and a load carrying endosseous implant at the light microscopic level*. There are many different endosteal implant systems available, and it is beyond the scope of this book to discuss all the systems and their various advantages and disadvantages. The Brånemark system, described here, is probably the best known and has been researched over the longest period demonstrating acceptable 15-year success rates. However, whatever the system used, radiology plays an essential role in preoperative treatment planning, postoperative follow-up and success evaluation.

The Brånemark system

This usually involves either a two-stage or a one-stage (non-submerged) surgical procedure followed by the restorative phase. Initially, in the two-stage technique the *fixture* is placed in vital bone ensuring a precision fit. The *cover screw* is screwed into the top of the *fixture* to prevent downgrowth of soft and hard tissue into the internal threaded area. The fixture is then left buried beneath the mucosa for 3–6 months. (It is important during this initial healing period to avoid loading the fixture although early loading protocols are being used in certain clinical circumstances.) The *fixture* is then surgically uncovered, the *cover screw* removed and the *abutment* (the transmucosal component) connected to the *fixture* by the *abutment screw*. An *hexagonal anti-rotation device* is incorporated into the top of the fixture. The *gold cylinder*, an integral part of the final restorative prosthesis, is finally connected to the abutment by the *gold screw*. A standard Brånemark implant is illustrated in Figure 21.1, although it should be emphasized that a variety of different abutments and connecting restorative elements, such as the EsthtiCone® and CeraOne® systems, are available for different clinical situations.

Main indications

Replacement of missing teeth in patients with:

- Healthy dentitions which have suffered tooth loss because of trauma
- Free-end saddles
- Developmentally missing teeth
- Remaining teeth not suitable as bridge abutments
- Severe ridge resorption making the wearing of dentures difficult
- Severe gag reflex

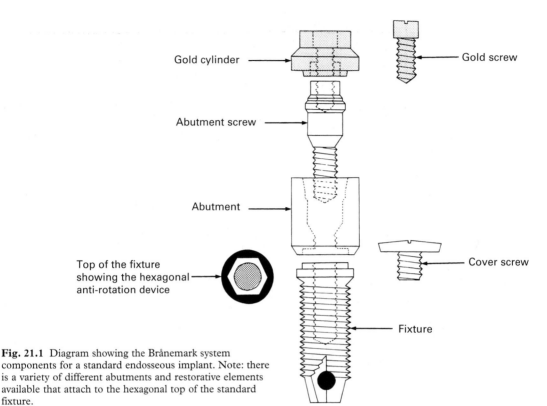

Gold cylinder

Gold screw

Abutment screw

Abutment

Cover screw

Top of the fixture
showing the hexagonal
anti-rotation device

Fixture

Fig. 21.1 Diagram showing the Brånemark system components for a standard endosseous implant. Note: there is a variety of different abutments and restorative elements available that attach to the hexagonal top of the standard fixture.

- Cleft palates and insufficient remaining teeth to support a denture/obturator
- Reconstruction following radical ablative jaw surgery
- A desire to avoid wearing a removable prosthesis.

Treatment planning considerations

Clinical examination

A thorough clinical examination using study casts, and overall evaluation of the patient are essential, as good case selection is imperative for the long-term success of implants. A multidisciplinary approach involving surgeons, prosthodontists and dental technicians is often adopted because of the many important factors that need to be taken into account, including:

- The patient's age, general health and motivation

- The condition and position of the remaining teeth (if present), including their occlusion
- The status of the periodontal tissues and the level of oral hygiene
- The condition — quality and quantity — of the edentulous mandibular or maxillary alveolar bone
- The condition of the oral soft tissues.

Radiographic examination

A comprehensive radiological assessment of the underlying mandible and/or maxilla is obviously necessary. The main investigations include:

- Dental panoramic tomographs occasionally supplemented with periapicals.
- Cross-sectional linear tomography programmes available with modern DPT machines.
- Multidirectional (e.g. spiral) cross-sectional tomography using for example the Scanora® (see Figs 21.2 and 21.3).

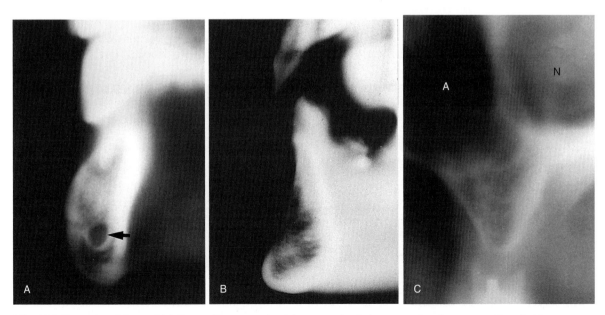

Fig. 21.2 Pre-implant assessment using the Scanora® multidirectional tomographic machine. **A** Dental panoramic tomograph of an edentulous patient showing various radiopaque localization markers (attached to the denture). **B** 4-mm cross-sectional (transverse) spiral tomographic images of the 321/ region. The location of each cross-sectional image is indicated on the panoramic radiograph. The radiopaque markers in the 3/ and 1/ regions are arrowed on both figures and are in focus on the tomographic slices.

Fig. 21.3 Examples of 4-mm thick Scanora® cross-sectional (transverse) spiral tomographs taken as part of pre-implant assessment. **A** Right mandibular premolar/molar region, showing the inferior dental canal (arrowed). **B** Midline of the mandible. **C** Right maxillary premolar region, also showing the antrum (A) and nasal cavity (N). All the images provide information on the quantity and quality of bone available.

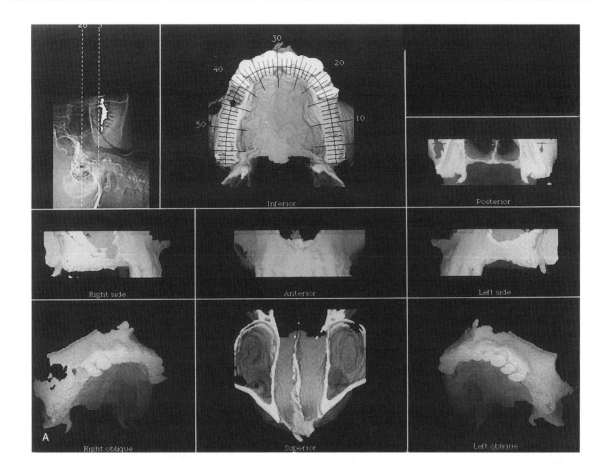

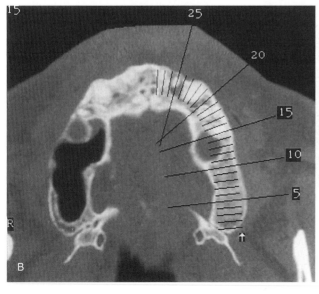

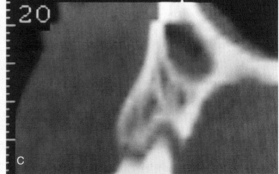

Fig. 21.4 Examples of CT images created by multiplanar reformatting used for pre-implant assessment in the maxilla. **A** Set of three-dimensional reconstructed images. **B** One axial slice showing the position of the various reconstructed cross-sectional images. (Kindly supplied by Dr A. Sidi.) **C** One reconstructed cross-sectional slice — number 20 from the axial slice shown in **B**.

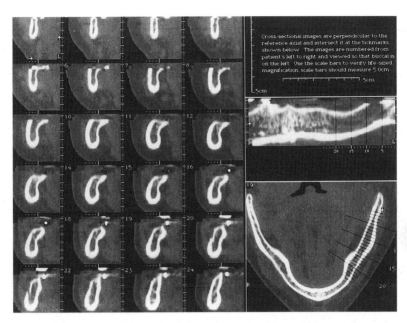

Fig. 21.5 Example of the three basic CT images created by multiplanar reformatting used for pre-implant assessment in the mandible showing a reconstructed panoramic view, an axial slice showing the position of the cross-sectional images and 24 of these reconstructed slices. (Kindly supplied by Mr R. Wilson.)

- CT. This usually involves about 30 axial scans per jaw, each 1.5 mm thick. This information can then undergo computer manipulation to produce reformatted cross-sectional, panoramic and three-dimensional reconstructed images, as shown in Figures 21.4 and 21.5.

- MRI. This offers the advantages of not using ionizing radiation and producing sections in any desired plane without reformatting as shown in Figure 21.6.

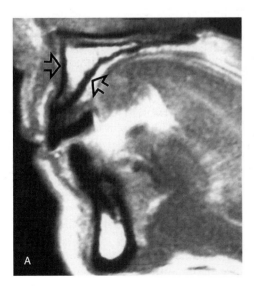

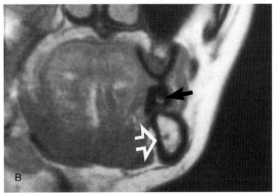

Fig. 21.6A Sagittal section MRI scan showing the bucco-palatal width and height of the edentulous anterior maxilla (arrowed). **B** Cross-sectional MRI image showing an edentulous left mandible (open arrow) and the stent containing the gadolinium marker (black arrow). The inferior dental canal is clearly evident. (Images kindly supplied by Mr Crawford Gray.)

These various radiographic investigations are used to show:

- The position and size of relevant normal anatomical structures, including the:
  — inferior dental canals
  — mental foramina
  — incisive or nasopalatine foramen and canal
  — nasal floor
- The shape and size of the antra, including the position of the antral floor and its relationship to adjacent teeth
- The presence of any underlying disease
- The presence of any retained roots or buried teeth
- The quantity of alveolar crest/basal bone, allowing direct measurements of the height, width and shape
- The quality (density) of the bone, noting:
  — the amount of cortical bone present
  — density of the cancellous bone
  — size of the trabecular spaces.

Important points to note

- Cross-sectional images (either multidirectional tomographs or CT) are essential to provide information on the width and quality of the alveolar bone. The two investigations complement one another. CT is recommended as the imaging modality of choice when information regarding the whole jaw or jaws is required, while multidirectional tomography is recommended for investigating small segments of a jaw.
- Some form of plastic stent containing radiopaque markers over the proposed implant sites or outlining the intended crown form (either custom-made or by modifying existing dentures) is often worn by the patient during the radiographic examination, to assist in accurate localization of cross-sectional images (see Fig. 21.2). Gadolinium markers are used with MRI (see Fig. 21.6B).
- The radiation dose from CT is quite high compared to conventional radiography and the investigation is usually more expensive. However, the information gathered can be manipulated and reformatted. In addition, the reconstructed images are usually life-size and CT can provide radiographic density values for cortical and cancellous bone. Specialized computer software such as SIM/Plant (Columbia Scientific Inc.) can be used with CT images to enable simulated implants to be inserted and viewed to assess size and angulation.
- The magnification on multidirectional cross-sectional tomographs varies from one machine to another, but for any particular unit it is fixed and uniform, e.g. Scanora® slices are all magnified by a factor of 1.7.

Postoperative evaluation and follow-up

Postoperative evaluation can be carried out immediately after surgery and usually after the initial 4–6 months healing period. Further clinical evaluation of the success or otherwise of the implant, including radiographic assessment, should be carried out on an annual basis for the first few years and then bi-annually. The radiographs used can be a combination of:

- Geometrically accurate paralleling technique periapicals. **Note**: The accuracy can be checked by examining the geometric thread pattern of the fixture
- Dental panoramic tomographs
- Digital radiographs
- Multidirectional cross-sectional tomographs.

Criteria for success

Ideally, implants should be evaluated against standardized success criteria and not simply assessed for their survival. Several *criteria for success* have been put forward over the years for the different implant systems. Those favoured by the author, and cited frequently in the literature, are those proposed by Albrektsson in 1986. These include:

1. That an individual, unattached implant is immobile when tested clinically.

2. That a radiograph does not demonstrate any evidence of peri-implant radiolucency.

3. That vertical bone loss be less than 0.2 mm annually following the implant's first year of service.

4. That individual implant performance be characterized by an absence of signs and symptoms such as pain, infection, neuropathies, paraesthesia or violation of the inferior dental canal.

5. That, in the context of the above, a success rate of 85% at the end of a 5-year observation period and 80% at the end of a 10-year period be the minimum criteria for success.

Radiographic evaluation (see Figs 21.7, 21.8 and 21.9)

Radiographs allow evaluation of criteria 2 and 3, but also are used to assess:

- The position of the fixture in the bone and its relation to nearby anatomical structures
- Healing and integration of the fixture in the bone

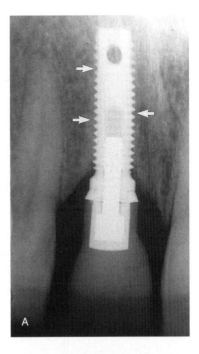

A

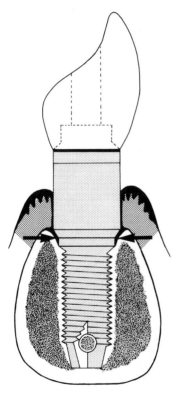

Fig. 21.7 Diagram showing (1) successful osseointegration — the bone/implant interface does not have fibrous tissue interposed, it is a direct contact and attachment between bone and the metallic implant surface, (2) minimal bone loss around the top of the implant, (3) no evidence of peri-implantitis and (4) a close fit of the abutment to the fixture (arrowed). These ideal features apply to the fixture and the surrounding tissues whatever type of abutment and restorative elements are chosen.

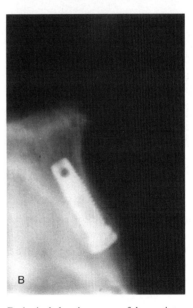

B

Fig. 21.8A Periapical showing successful osseointegration, 2 years after implant placement. Note the bone/implant interface (arrowed), there is no radiolucency in between. (Kindly supplied by Mr L. Howe.) **B** Cross-sectional spiral tomographic slice in the /1 region immediately after surgery showing the buccopalatal position and angulation of the implant.

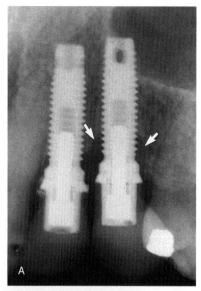

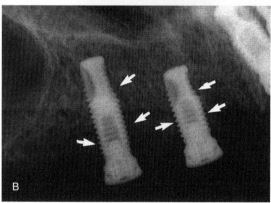

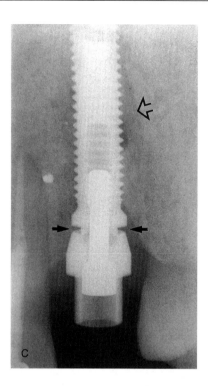

Fig. 21.9A Periapical showing vertical bone loss (arrowed) around the thread of the implant replacing /4, but virtually no bone loss around the implant replacing /3. **B** Periapical showing unsuccessful osseointegration. Note the radiolucent line between surrounding bone and the implants (arrowed), particularly mesially on the implant replacing 5/. **C** Periapical showing incorrect seating of the abutment on the fixture (solid arrows) and residual radiolucency from previous periapical area (open arrow). (Examples kindly supplied by Professor R. Palmer, Mr Saravanamuttu and Mr L. Howe.)

- The peri-implant bone level and any subsequent vertical bone loss — threaded fixtures allow easy measurement if radiographs are geometrically accurate
- Development of any associated disease, e.g. *perimplantitis*
- The fit of the abutment to the fixture
- The fit of the abutment to the crown/prosthesis
- Possible fracture of the implant/prosthesis.

Footnote

The limited nature of the information provided by conventional two-dimensional radiographs on the width or thickness of the alveolar bone cannot be overemphasized. Inadequate clinical and radiographic assessment of possible implant sites, before surgery, may lead to implant failure and more seriously, to temporary or permanent nerve damage and possible litigation.

22 Atlas of diseases and abnormalities affecting the jaws

Dental nurses should be aware of the more common diseases and important abnormalities that can affect the jaws. Detailed interpretative skills are not required, more the ability to recognise the abnormal. This chapter is therefore designed like an atlas to show examples of some of the conditions that have characteristic radio-graphic features. The lesions shown can be broadly grouped into:

- Developmental abnormalities
- Cysts
- Tumours – odontogenic and non-odontogenic
- Fibro-cemento-osseous lesions

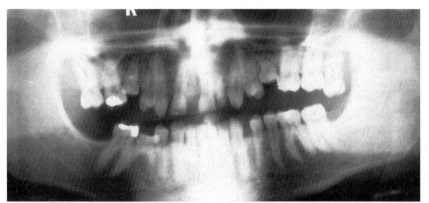

Fig. 22.1 Dental panoramic tomograph showing hypodontia

8	5	2	5
87	5		8

are congenitally missing and /2 is rudimentary and peg-shaped.

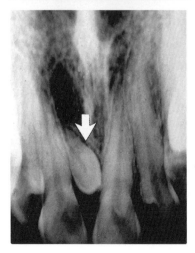

Fig. 22.2 Periapical showing a supernumerary or mesiodens (arrowed) between 1/1.

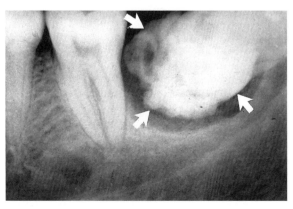

Fig. 22.3 Periapical showing a complex odontome, a disorganized mass of dental tissues in /7 region (arrowed).

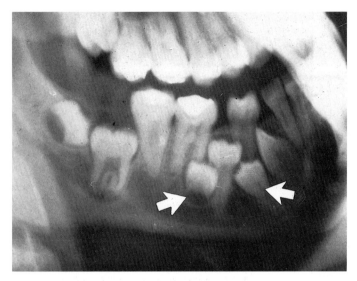

Fig. 22.4 Oblique lateral showing two supplemental lower premolars (arrowed) and a developing $\overline{9|}$.

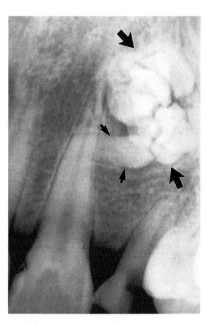

Fig. 22.5 Periapical showing a compound odontome in the anterior maxilla — several small discrete denticles are evident (arrowed) (right).

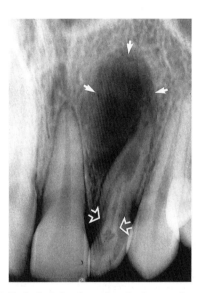

Fig. 22.6 Periapical showing a dens-in-dente or invaginated odontome involving $\underline{|2}$ (open arrows). There is an associated periapical area of infection (solid arrows) — a common occurrence with dens-in-dente.

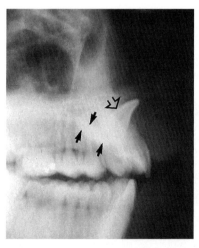

Fig. 22.7 Lateral view showing a dilacerated $\underline{|1}$. The crown (open arrow) and the root (solid arrows) are in different planes as a result of the near right angle bend in the root.

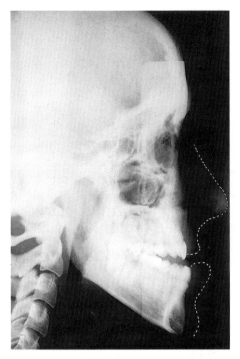

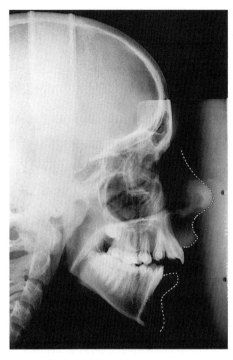

Fig. 22.8 True cephalometric lateral skull showing macrognathia (overgrowth of the mandible) in skeletal Class III. The soft tissue profile has been drawn in.

Fig. 22.9 True cephalometric lateral skull showing micrognathia (underdeveloped mandible) in skeletal Class II. The soft tissue profile has been drawn in.

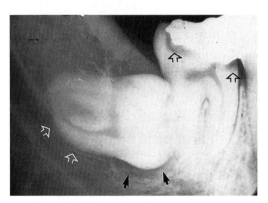

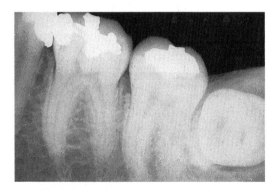

Fig. 22.10 Horizontally impacted $\overline{8}$. Note the pincer-shaped roots and their indentation of the upper margin of the inferior dental canal (open white arrows) and radiolucency beneath the crown (solid black arrows) caused by the follicle. In addition, note the carious lesions in $\overline{7}$ (open black arrows).

Fig. 22.11 Transversely positioned $\overline{8}$. The crown is viewed end-on. Note that the bucco/lingual obliquity of the tooth cannot be determined from this radiograph.

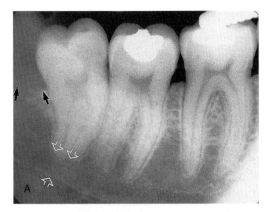

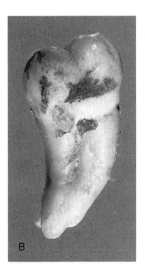

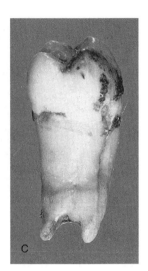

Fig. 22.12 A Slightly distoangularly impacted $\overline{8|}$. Note the extensive area of bone resorption distal to the crown (black arrows) caused by previous pericoronal infection. There is a radiolucent band across the tooth apex which is also hazy in outline (open white arrows) caused by the inferior dental canal, implying an intimate relationship. **B** The extracted $\overline{8|}$, viewed as in the radiograph from the buccal aspect. **C** The extracted tooth viewed from the distal aspect showing clearly the notching of the tooth apex by the inferior dental canal. This explains the radiolucent band across the apex — there is simply less tooth tissue in this zone, because of the position of the inferior dental canal. (Specimen and radiograph kindly supplied by Dr A. Sidi.)

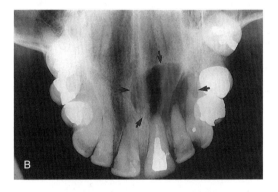

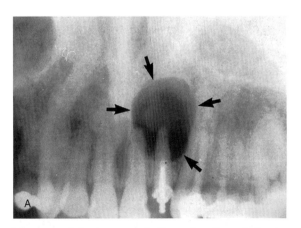

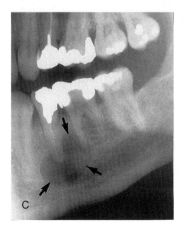

Fig. 22.13 A Static panoramic (Panoral) radiograph showing a typical radicular (dental) cyst (arrowed) associated with the non-vital $\underline{|2}$. **B** Upper standard occlusal showing a large radicular cyst associated with the root-filled $\underline{|1}$. **C** Part of a DPT showing a typical monolocular radicular cyst associated with the non-vital $\overline{|5}$.

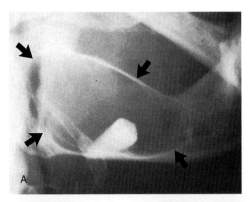

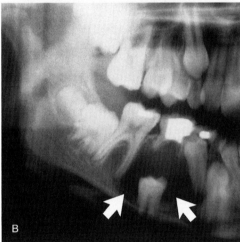

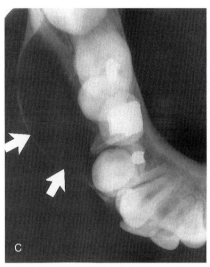

Fig. 22.14 A Oblique lateral of the right side of the mandible showing a typical circumferential dentigerous cyst (arrowed) associated with the unerupted and displaced $\overline{8/}$. **B** Part of a DPT showing a monolocular central dentigerous cyst (arrowed) associated with the unerupted and inferiorly displaced $\overline{5/}$. **C** Right side of a lower 90° occlusal of the same patient showing the typical buccal expansion (arrowed).

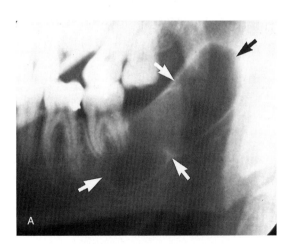

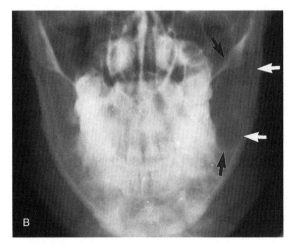

Fig. 22.15 A Oblique lateral of the left side of the mandible showing a typically extensive pseudolocular odontogenic keratocyst (arrowed) which has apparently developed instead of $/\overline{8}$. **B** PA jaws of the same patient showing that it has caused minimal mediolateral expansion (arrowed).

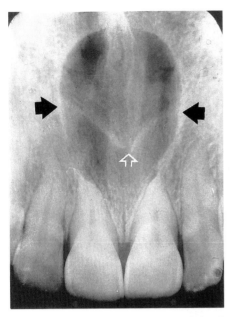

Fig. 22.16 Periapical showing a typical nasopalatine duct cyst (solid arrows) in the midline between the upper central incisors. Note the superimposed shadow of the anterior nasal spine (open white arrows) causing the cyst to appear heart-shaped.

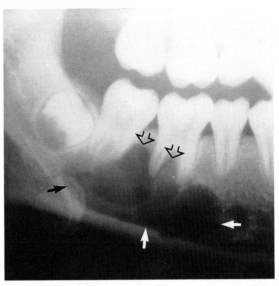

Fig. 22.17 Oblique lateral of the right side of the mandible of a teenager showing a typical solitary bone cyst (solid arrows) in the body of the mandible. Note the upper border arching up between the roots of the molar teeth (open arrows).

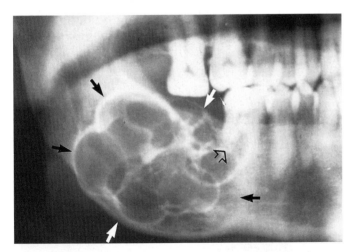

Fig. 22.18 Part of a DPT showing the typical multilocular appearance of a large ameloblastoma at the angle of the mandible, with extensive expansion (solid arrows) and resorption of adjacent teeth (open arrow).

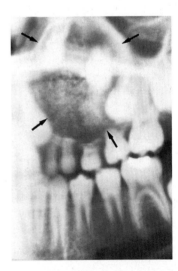

Fig. 26.19 Part of a DPT showing a monolocular adenomatoid odontogenic tumour in the anterior maxilla (arrowed) surrounding the unerupted /3. Internal calcification is evident.

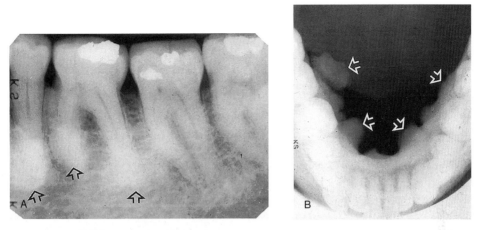

Fig. 22.20 A Periapical of /5678 showing ill-defined areas of radiopacity (arrowed) overlying the teeth. **B** Lower 90° occlusal of the same patient showing the large irregular exostoses (mandibular tori) on the lingual aspect of the mandible (arrowed).

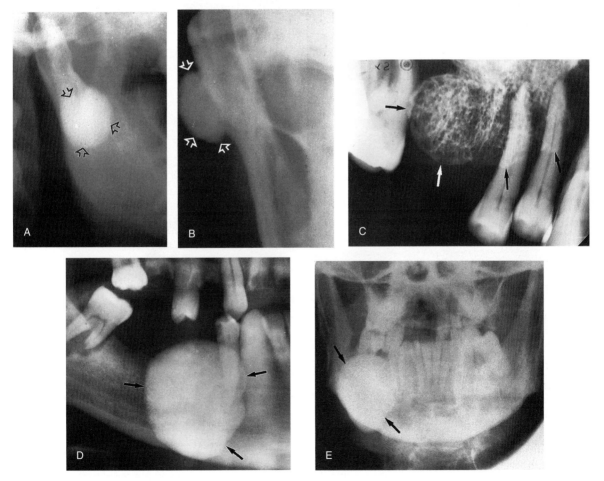

Fig. 22.21 A Oblique lateral of right ramus of the mandible showing a round radiopaque compact osteoma (arrowed). **B** Part of a PA jaws of the same patient showing the lesion (arrowed) arising from the lateral surface of the mandible confirming a periosteal osteoma. **C** Periapical showing a periosteal cancellous osteoma (arrowed). **D** Part of a DPT and **E** PA jaws of the same patient showing a very large endosteal compact osteoma (arrowed) in the body of the mandible.

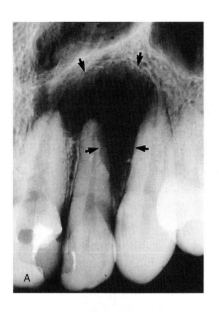

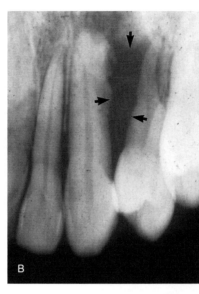

Fig. 22.22 **A** Periapical of /123 showing a poorly defined ragged area of radiolucency (arrowed) with resorption of the lateral aspect of /2 root. Biposy revealed an osteolytic osteosarcoma. **B** Periapical showing a similar smaller poorly defined area of bone destruction between /34 (arrowed) which was again shown to be an osteosarcoma.

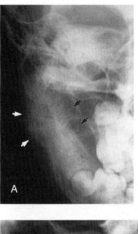

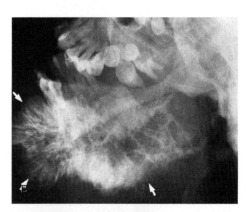

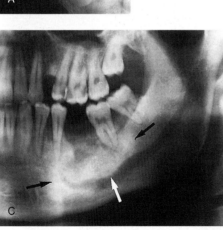

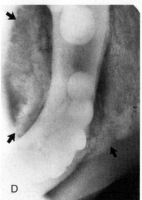

Fig. 22.23 **A** Right side of a PA jaws of a 7-year-old showing an osteosarcoma in the ascending ramus of the mandible. The *sunray* or *sunburst* appearance is evident medially and laterally (arrowed). **B** Oblique lateral showing a very extensive osteogenic osteosarcoma of the mandible with obvious *sunray* or *sunburst* bone formation. **C** Left side of a DPT showing an irregular, poorly defined area of radiopacity (arrowed) in the body of the mandible. **D** Lower 90° occlusal of the same patient showing extensive buccal and lingual abnormal bone formation (arrowed) of another osteogenic osteosarcoma.

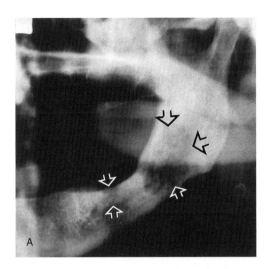

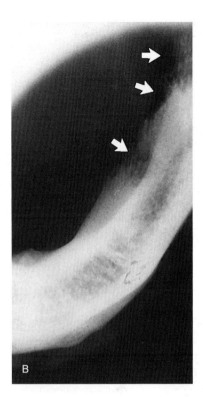

Fig. 22.24 A Part of a DPT of a patient who presented with a large squamous cell carcinoma on the left ventral surface of his tongue and the floor of his mouth. The radiograph shows two areas of poorly defined radiolucency (arrowed) with a ragged or *moth-eaten* appearance. **B** Left side of a lower 90° occlusal of the same patient showing the bony destruction (arrowed) of the lingual surface of the mandible as the soft tissue tumour invades the bone.

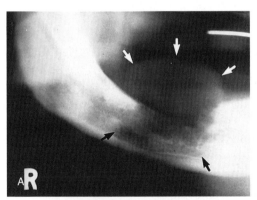

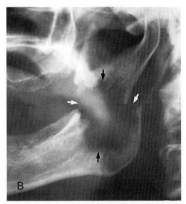

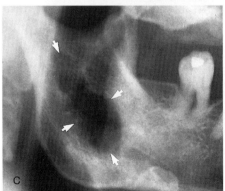

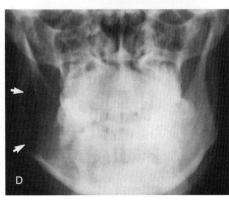

Fig. 22.25 A Right side of a DPT showing the typical destructive, *moth-eaten* radiolucency of a malignant lesion (black arrows). Overlying soft tissue involvement is also evident (white arrows). Subsequent investigation showed this to be a secondary metastatic tumour from the breast. **B** Left side of a DPT showing a large irregular destructive secondary metastatic tumour in the ascending ramus (black arrows). There is an associated pathological fracture (white arrows). **C** Right side of a DPT. **D** PA jaws of the same patient showing a poorly defined radiolucent secondary metastatic deposit, from the lung, presenting centrally in the ramus (arrowed).

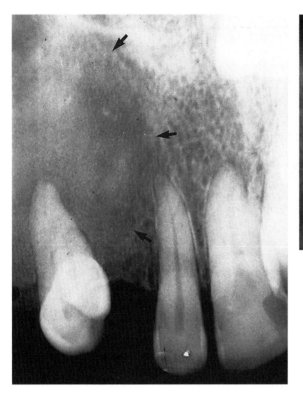

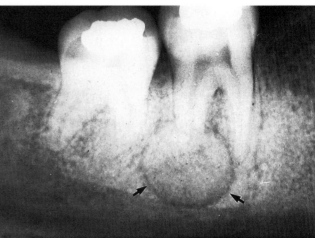

Fig. 22.27 Periapical showing the typical radiopaque mass at the apex of the $\overline{6/}$ of a benign cementoblastoma, the so-called *golf ball* appearance. The mass is attached to the root and has a thin radiolucent line around it (arrowed).

Fig. 22.26 Periapical of the upper right maxilla showing the generalized radiolucency with the fine internal trabeculation of monostostic fibrous dysplasia, giving a *ground glass* appearance. The almost imperceptible junction between abnormal and normal bone is arrowed.

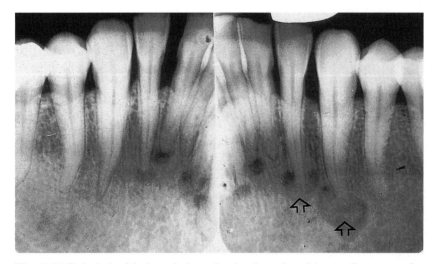

Fig. 22.28 Periapicals of the lower incisors showing the early and intermediate stages of periapical cemento-osseous dysplasia. Several, small, discrete radiolucencies are evident at the apices. The more mature lesions at the apices $/\overline{23}$ show evidence of internal calcification (open arrows).

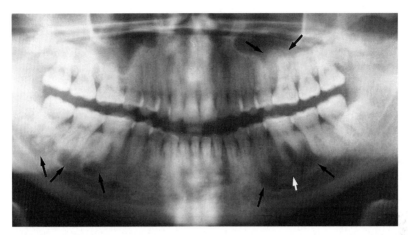

Fig. 22.29 Dental panoramic tomograph showing the multiple lesions (arrowed) of variable radiodensity of florid cemento-osseous dysplasia.

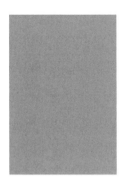

BIBLIOGRAPHY AND SUGGESTED READING

Part 1
Introduction (Ch. 1)

Coren S, Porac C, Ward LM 1979 Sensation and perception. Academic Press, New York

Cornsweet TN 1970 Visual perception. Academic Press, New York

Lindsay PH, Norman DA 1977 Human information and processing. 2nd edn. Academic Press, New York

Part 2
Radiation physics and equipment (Chs 2–5)

Armstrong SJ 1990 Lecture notes on the physics of radiology. Clinical Press, Bristol

Curry TS, Dowdey JE, Murry RC 1990 Christensen's physics of diagnostic radiology 4th edn. Lea and Febiger, Philadelphia

Graham DT 1996 Principles of radiological physics 3rd edn. Churchill Livingstone, Edinburgh

IPEM 1998 Recommended standards for the routine performance testing of diagnostic X-ray imaging systems. IPEM Report No. 771998

Mason RA, Bourne S 1998 A guide to dental radiography. 4th edn. Oxford University Press, Oxford

NRPB 1994 Guidelines on radiology standards in primary dental care. National Radiological Protection Board, Vol. 5, No. 3 1994

NRPB/DH 2001 Guidance notes for dental practitioners on the safe use of X-ray equipment.

Smith NJD 1989 Dental radiography. 2nd edn. Blackwell Scientific Publications, Oxford

Strather JW, Muirhead CR, Edwards AA et al 1988 Health effects models developed from the UNSCEAR report. National Radiological Protection Board, Chilton, NRPB-R226. HMSO, London

Sumner D, Wheldon T, Watson W 1991 Radiation risks: an evaluation. 3rd edn. The Tarragon Press, Glasgow

Tanner RJ, Wall BF, Shrimpton PC, Hart D, Bungay DR. Frequency of medical and dental X-ray examinations in the UK –1997/98. NRPB-R320 (2000), Chilton

Part 3
Radiation protection (Ch. 6)

Approved code of practice: the protection of persons against ionising radiation arising from any work activity. The ionising radiations regulations 1985. HMSO, London

Bury B, Hufton A, Adams J 1995 Radiation and women of childbearing potential. British Medical Journal 310:1022–23

FGDP(UK) 1998 Selection criteria for dental radiography. Royal College of Surgeons of England, London

Guidance notes for dental practitioners on the safe use of X-ray equipment 2001. NRPB/DoH, London

Health and Safety at Work, etc. Act 1974. HMSO, London

ICRP publication 60 1990 Recommendations of the International Commission on Radiological Protection. Annals ICPR 21. Nos 1–3. Pergamon Press, Oxford

Lecomber AR, Downes SL, Mokhtari M, Faulkner K 2000 Optimisation of patient doses in programmable dental panoramic radiography. Dentomaxillofacial Radiology 29:107–12

Napier ID 1999 Reference doses for dental radiography. British Dental Journal 186:8 392–396

NRPB 1994 Guidelines on radiology standards in primary dental care. National Radiological Protection Board, Vol. 5, No. 3 1994

NRPB 1999 Guidelines on patient dose to promote the optimisation of protection for diagnostic medical exposures. National Radiological Protection Board, Vol. 10, No. 1 1999

Ionising Radiations Regulations 1999. SI 1999 No 3232. HMSO, London

Ionising Radiation (Medical Exposure) Regulations 2000. SI 2000 No 1059. HMSO, London

Sharp C, Shrimpton JA, Berry RF 1998 Diagnostic medical exposures – Advice on Exposure to ionising radiation during pregnancy. Joint guidance from National Radiological Protection Board

White SC 1992 Assessment of radiation risk from dental radiography. Dentomaxillofacial Radiology 21:118–26

Part 4
Radiography (Chs 7–17)

British Orthodontic Society. Guidelines for the use of radiographs in clinical orthodontics 2001 2nd edn. London

de Lyre W, Johnson O 1995 Essentials of dental radiography for dental assistants and hygienists. 5th edn. Prentice-Hall, New Jersey

Haring IH, Jansen L 2000 Dental radiography-principles and techniques. 2nd edn. WB Saunders, Philadelphia

Horner K 1992 Quality assurance: 1 Reject analysis, operator technique and the X-ray set. Dental Update 19:75–80

Horner K 1992 Quality assurance: 2 The image receptor, the darkroom and processing. Dental Update 19:120–2

IPEM 1991 Quality assurance in dental radiology. IPEM report No.67

Jones ML, Oliver RG 1994 Walther and Houston's orthodontic notes. 5th edn. Butterworth-Heinemann, Oxford

Langland OE, Langlais RP 1997 Principles of dental imaging. Williams and Wilkins, Baltimore

Langland OE, Langlais RP, McDavid WD, Delbalso AM 1989 Panoramic radiology. Lea and Febiger, Philadelphia

Mason RA, Bourne S 1998 A guide to dental radiography. 4th edn. Oxford University Press, Oxford

McDonald F, Ireland AJ 1998 Diagnosis of the orthodontic patient. Oxford University Press, Oxford

NRPB/DH 2001 Guidance notes for dental practitioners on the safe use of X-ray equipment

Proceedings of the second symposium on digital imaging in dental radiology, Amsterdam 1992 Dentomaxillofacial radiology 21:179–221

Proceedings of the third symposium on digital imaging in dental radiology, Noorwijkerhout, The Netherlands 1995 Dentomaxillofacial radiology 24:67–106

Smith NJD 1989 Dental radiography. 2nd edn. Blackwell Scientific Publications, Oxford

The British standards glossary of dental terms BS 4492: 1983

White SC, Pharoah MJ 2004 Oral radiology principles and interpretation. 5th edn. CV Mosby, St. Louis

World Health Organisation. Quality assurance in diagnostic radiology 1982 Geneva WHO

Part 5
Radiology (Chs 18–31)

Albrektson T, Zarb GA 1989 The Branemark osseointegrated implant. Quintessence, Chicago

Brocklebank L 1996 Dental radiology (understanding the X-ray image). Oxford University Press

Browne RM, Edmondson HD, Rout PGJ 1995 Atlas of Dental and Maxillofacial Radiology. Mosby-Wolfe

FGDP(UK) 1998 Selection criteria in dental radiography. Royal College of Surgeons of England, London

Frommer HH 2001 Radiology for dental auxilaries. 7th edn. CV Mosby, St Louis

McMinn RMH, Hutchings and Logan BM 1999 Head and neck anatomy 2nd edn. Mosby-Wolfe, Edinburgh

Palmer RM 2000 A clinical guide to implants in dentistry. British Dental Association, London

Rudolphy MP, van Amerongen JP, ten Cate JM 1994 Radiopacities in dentine under amalgam restorations. Caries research 28:240–45

White SC, Pharoah MJ 2004 Oral radiology – principles and interpretation. 5th edn. CV Mosby, St. Louis

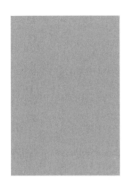

Index